"As a health-co... ... g more than to give my kids the very best foods to help them flourish. From day one, supplying nutritious and delicious superfoods will help create lifelong habits. Dana is a master, and I've trusted her expertise not only for my own books, but also in the foods I prepare in my own home. *First Bites* is a first choice for your infant or toddler."

—MARIO LOPEZ

"This accessible, sensible, and thoroughly modern take on nourishing your little one has just become my go-to baby gift for any new mom. These are tips and recipes befitting a new generation of healthy yet adventurous eaters. What a brilliant concept: baby food that isn't just nutritious—but also just plain delicious."

—KELLEY HEYWORTH,
editor of happyhealthykids.com

"Cooking creative, healthy meals for babies and toddlers can pose a challenge for busy parents. Dana does a wonderful job presenting easy tips and enticing recipes . . . I will be giving a copy of *First Bites* as a gift to my expecting friends and family members. It's a must-have book for every parent!"

—TOBY AMIDOR, MS, RD,
author of *The Greek Yogurt Kitchen*
and columnist for *Today's Dietitian*

"*First Bites* is a must-read for busy, health-conscious parents. Dana Angelo White not only explains exactly what you should feed your baby and why it's important, but she shares simple, delicious, and nutritious recipes that will make you excited to start cooking." —DR. KELLY MCNELIS, New Leaf Wellness

"This book is so perfect for new parents. And there's no better person to write it than registered dietitian Dana White who is not just a nutrition expert, but a mom of two herself . . . My only 'complaint' is that it wasn't available when I was a new parent trying to figure out the confusing world of feeding my own kids smart fuel for their growing bodies."

—CHRISTOPHER R. MOHR, PhD, RD,
owner of MohrResults.com

FIRST BITES

Superfoods for Babies and Toddlers

DANA ANGELO WHITE, MS, RD, ATC

A PERIGEE BOOK

A PERIGEE BOOK
Published by the Penguin Group
Penguin Group (USA) LLC
375 Hudson Street, New York, New York 10014

USA · Canada · UK · Ireland · Australia · New Zealand · India · South Africa · China

penguin.com

A Penguin Random House Company

Library of Congress Cataloging-in-Publication Data

White, Dana Angelo.
  First bites : superfoods for babies and toddlers / Dana Angelo White, MS, RD, ATC.
    pages cm
  "A Perigee Book."
  ISBN 978-0-399-17246-5 (paperback)
  1. Infants—Nutrition. 2. Toddlers—Nutrition. 3. Baby foods. I. Title.
  RJ216.W596 2015
  641.3'00832—dc23   2014040028

First edition: February 2015

PRINTED IN THE UNITED STATES OF AMERICA

10 9 8 7 6 5 4 3 2 1

Text design by Pauline Neuwirth

Most Perigee books are available at special quantity discounts for bulk purchases for sales promotions, premiums, fund-raising, or educational use. Special books, or book excerpts, can also be created to fit specific needs. For details, write: Special.Markets@us.penguingroup.com.

Contents

Introduction

F rom the moment your child is born you want to give them the best of everything. Every parent wants to provide nutritious and delicious things for their little ones to eat; the tricky part is deciding which foods are best and how to prepare them in a realistic amount of time. With so much conflicting nutrition info out there, parents can (and do) drive themselves bonkers, trying to make healthy choices.

By four to six months of age it is time to start introducing solids to your infant. From then on your goal should be to offer a wide variety of foods they will enjoy, while providing the nutrients they need to grow and thrive. However, many parents are often unsure of how to balance the right kinds of proteins, carbohydrates, healthy fats, and vitamins and minerals vital for proper growth and development. Plus, finding the time to prepare healthy meals can seem overwhelming, especially for new parents.

Recent nutrition research has found that most children fail to meet the recommendations for important nutrients like calcium, vitamin D, protein, fiber, and iron. According to the Academy of Nutrition and Dietetics, less than 50 percent of toddlers ages two to three consume the recommended daily amount of fruits and veggies. More surprising is a 2012 survey of parents that found that most had never received advice on feeding their toddlers. This lack of knowledge can have long-term effects on young growing bodies and minds. A study published in October 2013 discovered that poor nutrition during the first five years might also lead to behavioral problems.

I created *First Bites* with health-conscious parents in mind. I hope you can use this book as a quick and easy reference guide that you can keep on hand to whip up tasty and nutritious meals in no time. Family-centric recipes featuring fifty astoundingly nutritious and delicious superfoods are designed to help foster healthy eating habits and create a diet filled with fresh, minimally processed foods that are just as delicious as they are healthy. In this book, fruit and veggies take center stage in new and exciting ways, yet you will also learn to create healthy spins on classic kid favorites like mac and cheese, pizza, chicken fingers, and cupcakes.

· WHAT'S A SUPERFOOD? ·

"Superfood" is an abused term. Some less reliable sources on nutrition lead people to believe that any food dubbed "super" is magical, and one bite will cure anything. My definition is much different. For a food to reach super status, it must be delicious, beautiful, unprocessed, and bursting with nutrients. Bananas and brown rice are obvious super choices, but exposing tiny palates to more unique foods like quinoa and bison also offers a plethora of good nutrition plus some exciting flavors and textures to explore. My list of fifty foods represents a well-rounded group that is affordable, easy to find, and filled with the nutrients that growing bodies need more of. Incorporating these whole foods into your household will help promote growth, energy, strength, and brain power.

In addition to the fifty superfoods, the recipes in this book are made with *real* foods—each crafted with taste, nutrition, and palatability in mind. There are no artificial sweeteners or highly processed junk. I choose to use mostly natural sweeteners like honey and maple syrup but strongly believe that it is also OK to use regular old granulated sugar in moderation. Instead of chomping on candy and commercially baked goods in my house, we eat homemade frozen yogurt and cupcakes, made with a small amount of sugar.

There are two central themes of this book. First, a focus on the fifty superfoods, vibrant and exploding with flavor and nutrition. Second is a user-friendly guide (a handbook of sorts) for busy parents forever struggling to get healthy meals on the table.

To make this as effortless as possible, this book starts with a list of fifty foods along with a description of their nutrient content and health benefits. Each superfood listing also includes a list of the age-appropriate recipes where they are featured.

I've also included my best tips for grocery shopping, meal planning, and must-have kitchen tools. Recipe chapters are organized by food group (fruits and vegetables, grains, protein, and dairy and eggs). Each chapter is further divided into age-appropriate sections—six to twelve months, twelve to eighteen months, eighteen to twenty-four months, and two to three years to help parents make recipes that are best suited to the needs and preferences of their child as they grow. To wrap things up, the final chapter features menus for everything from family outings to weeknight playdates.

• NOTES FROM MY KITCHEN •

My kids aren't perfect eaters—far from it! But a lifelong love of food and culinary training and an advanced degree in nutrition has led me to one conclusion about feeding kids: what is most important is spending time together in the kitchen as a family. I did not write this book to be the nutrition "expert" or guru but to share recipes that my family loves, and I hope yours will too.

There is a huge behavior component to the way that we eat. Our preferences begin to shape from the moment we are born and continue to develop with time and experience. Learning what we like and dislike is an ever-changing process. Parents should remember this, embrace it, and not fight it.

Raising healthy and happy eaters takes trial and error. It is a marathon (maybe even an Ironman), not a sprint. But hopefully, as your little ones grow to be not so little anymore, they will develop a healthy and happy relationship with food.

Like I said, my kids aren't perfect. They have their likes and dislikes, and even with all that I have learned, there are days when my husband and I break all the rules. No matter what, we always make the extra effort not to fight with them over food. To make the family table a positive experience even on the days when the kids are driving us up the wall. Between my two daughters I have almost seven years of experience feeding in "the trenches." I used the same feeding strategies with both, and they could not be more different. One loves any and all fruits and vegetables and would literally eat them all day long. Meat, on the other hand, is not her favorite no matter how it is prepared. My other daughter is all about meat. From lamb chops to fish—she always wants more. She is much more selective when it comes to veggies, with a small number of acceptable options on her list. They both loved eggs, then decided they hated them, then loved them again—a roller coaster of drama, that's what little girls are made of in and out of the kitchen. There is one characteristic that they do share: they are (almost) always willing to try new things. They change every minute, and I embrace the excitement that comes along with their naturally dynamic nature.

In this book, I hope to share my knowledge, experience, and tips. I grew up loving food. From as early as I can remember I was sitting on the kitchen counter, observing, mixing, sprinkling, and learning from my parents. Taking it all in. My parents weren't chefs, but they both came from families who loved to cook. They instilled their love of food and cooking in my brother and me without even trying.

Since my days working and creating on the kitchen counter, my love of food has led to a career in nutrition, which has only further inspired my passion: carrying on the family tradition of sharing, appreciating, and loving delicious food. In a funny way I've been preparing to write this book forever. These are the meals we eat in my house every day—adults included! Family-centric, quick cooking that is never overly complicated. Fresh, easy, delicious, and healthy. The superfoods are our staple ingredients, and together the family explores the variety of these key foods. When my kids drag the step stool up to the counter yelling

"Can I help?" it only motivates me to create more recipes that we can explore together. Some of these recipes will be hits, others will fail miserably, but I am proud that so far my girls love to cook and love to eat. They have an education about food and where it comes from. They easily identify superfoods, like butternut squash, kale, edamame, and quinoa. They are no strangers to the garden, and our local farmer is a rock star in their eyes. So as far as I'm concerned, I'm doing my job.

1

What Growing Bodies Need

During the first three years, the rate of growth is more rapid than any other time in life. To support all this growth, kids need lots of nutrient-rich calories. The demand for vitamins and minerals is incredibly high, and some of these are easier to come by in the typical diet than others.

Dietary supplements may be an option for some children, but in general, food should always come first. Work with your pediatrician and a registered dietitian to determine your child's specific needs. Either way, make sure there are more of these five nutrients in their diet.

· CALCIUM ·

Function

Calcium is responsible for the proper growth and development of teeth and bones as well as muscle contraction and nerve conductivity.

Needs

Children ages newborn to three require between 200 and 700 milligrams of calcium per day.

Sources

Calcium can be found in dairy products like milk (300 milligrams in one cup), cheese, yogurt, and ice cream. It is also added to some brands of orange juice, tofu, and breakfast cereals. Other sources include almonds, broccoli, and leafy green vegetables like spinach and kale.

Deficiency in Children

In severe cases calcium deficiency can cause weakened teeth and bones. Poor intake of calcium during childhood can affect bone health later in life, and when kids grow older they may be at greater risk for bone fractures and osteoporosis.

· VITAMIN D ·

Function

The body needs vitamin D to absorb calcium and mineralize bone. Vitamin D is also important for immunity and healthy muscles.

Needs

Vitamin D is measured in international units (IU). Children ages newborn to three require 400 to 600 IU per day.

Sources

Vitamin D is found in a relatively small number of foods, which may make it difficult for some kids to get enough. Mothers who exclusively breastfeed are encouraged to give babies vitamin D supplement drops during the first six to twelve months. From food it can be found in fatty fish (like salmon and tuna), egg yolks, and fortified foods like milk, orange juice, some cuts of pork, and some brands of yogurt. There are 40 IU in a glass of milk and about 20 IU in one egg yolk.

Humans are able to make some of their own vitamin D with the skin's exposure to sunlight, but production varies on where you live and the time of year. Since there are plenty of other good reasons to keep the kids out of the sun (and slather on the sunblock), focusing on food should be a priority.

Deficiency in Children

In children, a lack of vitamin D can cause rickets, a rare but serious condition where the bones become weak and pliable. Children who suffer from rickets often have impaired growth, malformed teeth, and bowed legs.

· OMEGA-3 FATS ·

Function

Omega-3 fatty acids are forms of healthy, polyunsaturated fats. They play an important role in circulation and neurological function. One form in particular, referred to as DHA, is beneficial for pregnant women, infants, and children, contributing to healthy skin, vision, neurological development, and cognitive function.

Needs

There are no established government recommendations for omega-3 intake for babies and children, but pediatricians recommend somewhere between 400 and 700 milligrams a day for infants and children ages newborn to three years.

Sources

In addition to prenatal vitamins, moms are encouraged to take omega-3 supplements from fish oil during pregnancy and for breastfeeding. As infants grow there are additional options to take in this important nutrient. Some brands of milk and many brands of infant formula have DHA added.

Fatty fish like salmon and tuna are wonderful sources of omega-3, but since these aren't the most popular food choices for many children, flaxseeds, walnuts (barring a nut allergy), egg yolks, and fortified foods like cereals, milk and yogurt, and some varieties of jarred baby foods also have DHA added.

Deficiency in Children

Kids who don't get enough omega-3 may be at a greater risk for learning deficits and possibly behavioral issues.

· IRON ·

4

Function

Iron is one of the most important minerals for children and adults. It allows red blood cells to deliver oxygen to tissues and helps form enzymes that allow for all kinds of necessary body processes.

Needs

Requirements for iron shift with periods of growth. Children require 11 milligrams a day up to age twelve months, and then between ages one and three requirements decrease to 7 milligrams per day.

Sources

Iron can be found in plant-based foods like beans, raisins, lentils, spinach, tofu, and whole grain cereals as well as animal foods like red meat, poultry, tuna, and pork. Ideally it is best to eat a combination of both plant and animal sources of iron to maximize absorption.

Deficiency in Children

Not getting enough iron can lead to iron-deficiency anemia. Symptoms include headache, pale skin, fatigue, decreased appetite, shortness of breath, and decreased immunity. Deficiencies may also be accelerated by an excessive amount of calcium intake; kids who overconsume milk may be at greater risk.

· PROBIOTICS ·

Function

Probiotics are healthy bacteria that keep the digestive system working properly. Getting enough can be very helpful for children with food intolerances or who are prone to other gastrointestinal conditions like diarrhea and reflux.

Needs

Like omega-3 fats, there are no established guidelines for probiotic intake. What is most important with

5

probiotics is that intake is consistent and a regular fixture in the diet. Occasional consumption is not going to have the desired effects.

Sources

Children's probiotic supplements exist, but in many cases, natural food sources should be parents' first choice. You will find these healthy bacteria in yogurt and kefir (a cultured milk product) as well as sourdough bread and fermented foods like miso. There are also some naturally existing probiotics in breast milk, and infant formulas are often fortified.

Deficiency in Children

Bouts of diarrhea, illnesses, or taking antibiotics tend to wipe out much of the healthy bacteria along the digestive tract, making children deficient in what they need for normal digestion. Taking probiotics can help repopulate the digestive tract with what it needs to stay healthy.

• FEEDING KIDS •

The First Six Months: Life Before Solids

There are no meal plans for the first four to six months of a baby's life. This is the time for an all-liquid diet. Nutrition comes from breast milk or formula, because an infant's digestive tract is too immature to handle much else. But things get more exciting when they are in the four- to six-month-old range.

Introducing Solid Foods

Babies cannot say, "Hey, Mom, give me some of that!" When they are ready to try solids there are several cues parents can look out for. Look for these signs somewhere around four to six months:

- Increase in appetite
- Ability to sit up with minimal assistance (can sit in a high chair)
- Head control—can hold head up independently
- Interest in food—looking, smelling, reaching

How to Introduce New Foods

New foods should be introduced independently. It is the easiest way to know if your child has an adverse reaction to a particular food. When introducing a new food, give it four to seven days to rule out any adverse reactions before moving on to something else or mixing with another food. Once you start to incorporate mixed foods, like a combo of meats with vegetables, be sure only one new food (if any) is part of the mixture.

Rash, vomiting, skin changes, hives, diarrhea, even increased fussing and spitting up may be indications that the food is not being comfortably digested.

Don't be deterred by a snarling face or unpleasantly puckered puss; a lot of time this is just a normal reaction to a foreign texture or flavor.

It has been well documented that it may take up to ten or more exposures to a new food before a child can truly determine if they like it or not. Parents often make the mistake of striking foods off the list of options, assuming their child does not like it, when they really just needed more of a chance to get used to it.

7

Age-Appropriate Foods from 6 Months to 3 Years

Rice and Other Grains

Dehydrated rice cereal is often the first solid food an infant will try. Rice-based foods are typically offered early on because they have a mild flavor, a soft texture, and a low risk of allergic reaction. Once rice is tolerated comfortably, move on to other grains like oatmeal and barley. Dry Cheerios (plain), breads, and pastas can start to be introduced around the seven- or eight-month mark. As children approach one year of age, they can tolerate more complex dishes such as grains pureed with fruits, vegetables, dairy, or protein.

Fruits and Vegetables

Some experts recommend starting with veggies instead of fruit out of concern that the sweetness of fruit may outshine the appeal of vegetables, but I always started with applesauce. Basic fruit and vegetable purees, thinned out to the proper consistency, are easy to make and loaded with nutrition. Switching back and forth between fruits and vegetables is a nice way to offer purees and diversify flavor offerings. After a few months, your little one will develop an impressive repertoire of produce to enjoy. Here is a suggested order for introduction:

- Apples, pears, bananas
- Carrots, butternut squash, sweet potatoes
- Peaches, apricots, plums
- Peas, avocados, green beans, spinach, beets, potatoes

Dairy

Cow's milk is not recommended for babies until they reach one year of age, but some dairy products can be introduced sooner. Experiment with whole milk yogurt and cheese somewhere between eight and ten months. If the yogurt is fruit flavored, make sure your child has already been introduced to that type of fruit. As for cheese, mild flavors like American, Monterey Jack, mild cheddar, and ricotta are a good place to start.

Eggs

Egg whites pose a higher risk of allergic reaction, so try a cooked egg yolk first, somewhere around eight to ten months. As infants approach age one, give egg whites a try. Once any potential reactions have been ruled out, it's a go for whole eggs.

Meat and Fish

Purees of meats like chicken, turkey, pork, lamb, and even beef and bison are typically well tolerated. Since at this stage your child's teeth are limited (or nonexistent), puree well to prevent choking.

As their tiny palates advance, make coarsely pureed concoctions of meats, vegetables, and grains. Ground meat recipes like burgers, meatballs, and meat loaf are great options and can be cut into easier-to-eat finger food.

Fish like cod and salmon may be acceptable before a baby turns one year old, but the strong flavor often proves to be too much for most tiny palates. Allow your child to try it in small amounts as they grow. Shellfish like shrimp carry a higher risk of allergy, so proceed more cautiously; consider waiting until your child is older than one year or possibly longer if shellfish allergies or numerous other food allergies run in the family. If in doubt, consult your pediatrician.

9

Water and Juice

As babies learn to navigate the kitchen table, they should also be getting their hands on a sippy cup. Try giving water (in the proper cup, of course). Babies are still getting plenty of fluid from their bottles, but it's good to get some practice. Juice can be introduced at or after six months, but keep the portions modest (approximately four ounces a day). Serve in a cup (instead of a bottle) diluted with water. Children who take in excessive amounts of juice pile up the calories, and have less interest in table foods and a greater risk of cavities.

SUGGESTED AGES FOR INTRODUCTION OF FOODS

AGE	GRAINS	FRUITS & VEGETABLES	EGGS	DAIRY	PROTEIN
Six months	Rice, oatmeal, barley	Apples, pears, bananas			
Eight to nine months	Cheerios, pasta, bread	Avocados, squash	Yolk	Yogurt, cheese	Beef, pork, poultry
Twelve months	Toast	Greens	Whites	Milk	
Twelve to eighteen months	Pizza, baked goods	Strawberries	Whole eggs	Ice cream	Fish
Eighteen to twenty-four months	Bagels		Omelets	Smoothies and shakes	
Two to three years	Sandwiches		Quiche		Shellfish, peanut butter*

*Since peanut butter has a high risk of allergic reaction, work with your pediatrician to decide when it might be best to introduce to your child.

Common Food Allergies and Sensitivities

Food allergies and intolerances are not the same thing, and it is important to know the differences. Food allergies involve an adverse immune system reaction that affects numerous organ systems; in the worst cases they can be life threatening. Less severe symptoms may include upset stomach, nausea, vomiting, diarrhea, numbness, tingling, hives, and rash. A food intolerance involves compromised digestion and may have similar stomach symptoms but does not risk a life-threatening condition. In many cases, children with food intolerances may be able to eat small amounts of problem food comfortably. Children may outgrow these conditions with age as their digestive and immune systems mature. Children under three are most at risk for allergies and intolerances to milk, eggs, and peanuts. Allergies and intolerances to tree nuts (such as almonds, pistachios, and walnuts), fish, and shellfish are also possible. Always be on the lookout for out-of-the-ordinary reactions to foods. If you suspect your child has a food allergy or intolerance, get your pediatrician involved. They will help determine whether a referral to an allergist is needed.

If your child suffers from an allergy or intolerance, they obviously have to steer clear of certain foods. The great news is there are many alternative options readily available.

No-No Foods for Little Ones

In addition to potential allergens, there are a few other foods parents should be mindful of to help keep kids on a path to healthy eating. Some are serious choking hazards; others carry potentially harmful food-borne pathogens.

> **Choking hazards:** hot dogs, sausages, raw carrots, whole nuts, popcorn, grapes, cherry tomatoes, large spoonfuls of peanut butter, tough/chewy meats[*]

---

[*] Children may be able to enjoy some of these foods as long as they are cut up appropriately.

Potentially contaminated foods: honey, agave, raw milk, and other unpasteurized dairy and eggs

A child's immature immune system is not equipped to fight off potential pathogens. Honey may carry botulism spores, and unpasteurized ("raw") dairy may be contaminated with food bugs like salmonella and listeria. Wait until children are one year old to have honey, and avoid raw dairy throughout childhood.

Picky Eaters

I've been interviewing experts about dealing with picky eaters for years, and there are times when all that I have learned goes out the window! Do your best, and when all else fails, take a deep breath and let it go. Don't get up and make something different. Let your child take ownership and decide not to eat—they won't starve to death if they skip dinner one night. Allow them to have some of the control; it will empower them. Believe it or not they will (almost always) come around.

TRY TO

- Lead by example—parents have to be willing to eat and try things too.
- Offer a combination of foods your child likes along with things that may be a bit outside their comfort zone.
- Have a discussion about where food comes from.
- Get to the farmers' market or plant a garden.
- Make mealtime fun—eat, talk, share.
- Prepare meals together.

TRY NOT TO

- Freak out!
- Get noticeably frustrated.
- Fight over meals.
- Use dessert or other food as a reward.
- Insist that your child eat everything on their plate.

· FOOD PREPARATION AND STORAGE TIPS ·

Strategies for Meal Planning

A little planning can go a long way. Sit down for a few minutes over the weekend and map out the meals you want to make. Consider your schedule; when are you working late that week versus when you have time to cook more-involved meals. To make things easier on myself, I follow a simple framework for weeknight dinners. Specifics can change with the seasons, but using these tips helps take some of the guesswork out of the daily burning question—what do I make tonight?

- 1 day vegetarian
- 1 day chicken (grilled in the summer, roasted in the winter)
- 1 day fish
- 1 day low prep/no prep (from the freezer or slow cooker)
- 1 day (Friday night) pizza

13

Grocery Shopping: Saving Money and Getting It All Done

I prefer certain grocery stores for meat and fish and others for things like snacks and produce, but who has time to go to three stores each week? In the summer months I also like to get out to the farmers' market to take advantage of all the locally grown offerings. You *can* make it easier. Use these strategies to help get it all done:

- Use a grocery delivery program for weekly staples like bananas, milk, and paper towels. Most have a delivery fee, but you can actually save money by paying attention to per-unit pricing and reducing impulse purchases.
- Pick one local farmers' market to visit a week (and bring the kids). If you can't find one near you, look into joining a CSA where you can get a weekly delivery of local foods.
- Alternate weeks at other stores—stock up when you can to save money and time.

Stocking a Healthy Pantry

It is a lot easier to cook healthy meals if you've got the right ingredients on hand. Here are ten pantry staples to always have on hand:

1. Pasta—whole grain and regular
2. Canned tomatoes
3. Honey or maple syrup
4. Rolled oats
5. Flours—all-purpose and whole wheat pastry flour
6. Whole grain cereals

7. Canned beans
8. Rice vinegar
9. Unsweetened cocoa powder
10. Mini dark chocolate chips

Storage: Using the Freezer

I love my freezer (freezers—I have an extra in the garage). Storing food in the freezer allows me to have weeknight dinners at the ready and hold on to the flavors of summer during the winter months.

For best results, make sure your freezer is at the proper temperature and use specially designated freezer bags and containers to keep foods fresh. Save time and money by freezing the following items:

- Sliced bread (toast to defrost)
- Prepared trays of meals like chicken Parm and mac and cheese
- Oven fries (peel, slice, and blanch potatoes; drain and freeze—place in oven from freezer)
- Baby food purees in small containers and ice cube trays
- Berries (clean and dry; place in an even layer on a sheet pan; freeze, then store in a bag)
- Cooked pancakes (microwave to defrost)
- Raw balls of cookie dough
- Peeled bananas for smoothies
- Prepared pesto in ice cube trays
- Soups, stews, tomato sauce, and chili

· NUTRITION POINTERS FOR PARENTS ·

I know an amazing network of parents. Whether it's about napping, footwear, potty training, or eating, we all share our experiences and work together to help. Here are just a few of the questions that have come up about feeding and nutrition.

Q: I follow a vegan diet, but my kids eat some meat. What is the truth about soy? Is there such a thing as too much? Does it affect adults and kids differently?

A: The soy issue is a buzzy topic, and I am asked about it frequently! I have researched it a lot and so far can't find any reliable evidence to support that it would be dangerous for kids or adults in the amounts that they typically eat. Soy made the list of superfoods—twice—edamame and tofu. It's an excellent protein source; it has all the same protein building blocks that animal protein does, without the cholesterol and unhealthy fats. I recommend choosing organic soy products the majority of the time.

Q: When you are transitioning to table food, what does a day of complete nutrition look like? How much should babies be eating table food?

A: Until babies are one year old, their primary source of nutrition is from breast milk or formula. *But* you start table foods early to help get them physically and behaviorally used to eating all the different types of solids. How much will vary for every child, but ideally by twelve months of age, they are comfortable with fruits, veggies, cheese, yogurt, cereals, bread, pasta, and meats. How much is really up to them—if the table foods seem to be satisfying them, you can back off on some of the bottle feedings.

As you know, once allergies have been ruled out, they can switch to cow's milk around age one as well.

Somewhere around the one-year mark, they should be comfortable with enough table foods to have three meals a day in addition to two or three bottles (most likely in the morning and evening). One of those bottles may eventually turn into a table food snack. By age three, they are typically off the bottles and on a schedule of three meals and two(ish) snacks a day.

Some ideas for a one-year-old:

Breakfast: fruit, toast or pancake, maybe some yogurt

Lunch: pasta, or a cut-up sandwich and some soup (yogurt or fruit could go here too)

Dinner (similar to lunch): pasta, rice, protein, vegetables (whatever the family is having)

17

Q: What do I do if I can't get my kids to drink milk—without chocolate in it?!

A: Such a popular question! We made a rule at my house—milk with dinner and two nights a week it can be chocolate. If it's chocolate milk, then fruit for dessert (no other options)—this has seemed to create a nice balance. And if it's been a sugar-filled day, I put the kibosh on it immediately. If they really don't like it or have trouble digesting it, dairy-free alternatives like soy, almond, and coconut milk might be worth trying; they are fortified to have the same amount of calcium and vitamin D as cow's milk. If all else fails, homemade chocolate milk allows you to control the amount of added sugar. Better it come from something with a lot of nutrients (like milk) than from candy and other junk food.

Q: My kids like to "snack" throughout the day and end up eating smaller meals—is this acceptable the way it is for grown-ups?

A: It is—as long as the snacks are healthy ones and they are still eating meals. Focus on superfoods like apples, berries, yogurt, cheese, peanut butter, and whole grains. Snacking is vital for keeping energy levels high (just like for adults). It's just our job to keep an eye on their snacking. We've all been there when they snacked too much and don't want an actual meal—as long as this doesn't happen all the time, you're in good shape.

Q: My kids are fairly thin and typically in the lower percentile for their height/weight at our checkups. What can I do to "fatten" them up? Milk shakes, etc.?

A: The occasional milk shake is totally fine, but if weight gain is warranted, you want them to gain the right kind of weight. High-calorie superfoods are the way to go—peanut butter, cheese, granola, smoothies with fruit and yogurt, even dishes like spaghetti and meatballs—all good!

Q: My kids always want juice! How much is too much?

A: Try to cap it at four ounces a day—tops! Always choose 100 percent fruit juice and dilute with water most of the time (juice boxes will happen, but dilute with water when using cups). If water isn't cutting it for them, try flavoring it up by adding citrus, melon, berries, whatever they like—even a splash of plain seltzer water or adding an ice cube might add the excitement they want.

Q: Is organic really a better option and worth the extra cost?

A: There's no need to buy all organic superfoods. Organic can be better, but it is not always worth the extra money. I get as much as I can at the farmers' market (doesn't have to be organic if it's that local). When at the grocery store I rely on the Environmental

Working Group's Dirty Dozen and Clean Fifteen to help me decide what's worth it. For example, apples tend to carry a high level of pesticide residues, so buying organic is a good choice. On the other hand, superfoods like avocados and sweet potatoes tend to be much less troublesome. Learn more at ewg.org/foodnews.

Q: Do I need to worry about sodium in my child's diet?

A: Sodium is an important nutrient for a wide variety of body functions including fluid balance and muscle contraction. Little bodies *need* sodium but only about 1,000 milligrams per day; check labels to make sure your kids aren't going overboard. As a general rule, the more whole foods (and less processed ones) in your child's diet, the less you have to worry about all that added sodium.

Q: My son has an atrocious diet. He eats very few foods. No meats, no veggies, one fruit. I just go with it hoping that one day he will change; I don't want to scar him when it comes to mealtime. Any advice to help?

A: I wish I had an easy answer, but there is none. But you are not alone! What I can say is don't give up. Keep trying to introduce new things to him. It can take ten or more exposures to a food for a child to truly determine they aren't a fan—and even

20

after that, they may change their mind a few years down the road. Look at the foods he is currently choosing from and see where you can make small changes. Fighting about it certainly won't help, but turning a blind eye and hoping he will change might not either. You can't force him, but you can provide the tools. As you know, kids like to take ownership of things; see if you can channel that into the kitchen. Allow him to participate in the shopping and prep. Start with the foods he will eat, and then explore some new things together.

Q: My child has a peanut allergy; he refuses to try the almond or sun butter.

A: I'm a huge fan of soy nut butter; it has a better texture. Add some honey and cinnamon for extra flavor. Thankfully most schools are nut-free, so all parents are in the same boat for lunches. Cream cheese and jelly has been popular for my girls' lunch boxes lately.

21

2

The Superfood Index and Must-Have Kitchen Tools

T here are a lot of things that can make a food "super." Nutrition is of course important, but so are things like variety, taste, and seasonality. Encouraging a diet rich in superfoods helps kids grow to love healthy foods *and* know and appreciate where they come from. These fifty foods contain the nutrients that growing bodies need, and provide them in the most colorful and tastiest of ways. Superfoods also don't have to be expensive or hard to find. All of these items are readily available at the local farmers' market or grocery store.

Here's my list of amazing superfoods along with some creative uses, age-appropriate guidelines, and recipes where they are featured. In the recipe chapters, all superfoods are identified in **bold**.

23

· 1. APPLES ·

Often a first fruit for babies to try, apples are full of fiber, vitamin C, and antioxidants. Little ones love apples for snacking or whirled into applesauce—a naturally sweet treat. Take the kids apple picking so they can see exactly where these gorgeous fruits come from.

WAYS TO ENJOY
- Sliced and dipped in yogurt
- Baked with cinnamon
- Pressed in a grilled cheese sandwich

Recipes: *Perfect Applesauce, Slow-Cooker Pulled Pork*

· 2. AVOCADOS ·

Avocados contain heart-healthy monounsaturated fats as well as vitamin C, vitamin K, folate, and potassium. This creamy green fruit (yes, it's technically a fruit) also contains lutein, a photochemical that benefits the development of healthy eyes, skin, and hair. Little ones love guacamole—get them started around seven or eight months of age. It gets a little messy, but it's totally worth it!

WAYS TO ENJOY
- Mixed into salsa
- Mashed as a sandwich spread
- Diced and sprinkled over rice

Recipe: *Guac for All Ages*

• 3. BANANAS •

Often used as one of the very first solid foods for babies, bananas provide vitamins and minerals like vitamin B6 and potassium—both vital for healthy muscles. The naturally soft texture and sweet flavor puts them at the top of the favorites list for both kids and parents. Bananas are also high in soluble fiber, which may constipate some infants, so proceed with caution when introducing this tasty fruit.

WAYS TO ENJOY
- Frozen and blended into a creamy treat
- Baked into breads and muffins
- Dipped in chocolate and frozen on a stick

Recipes: *Roasted Bananas with Cinnamon, Banana "Ice Cream," Maddy's Creamy Dreamy Banana Shake, Mango-Banana Almond Milk Smoothie, Grape Salsa, Banana Chocolate Chip Bread, Spoonable Smoothie, Yogurt Sundaes*

• 4. BEANS •

Packed with fiber and protein, beans are soft (easy on the gums) and appealing as finger food. Canned or dried, you'll find lots of other nutrients, including calcium, zinc, and iron. Beans can promote a gassy stomach for kids (just like they do for some adults), so consider waiting until they are closer to eight months and introduce them gradually.

25

WAYS TO ENJOY

- Mashed into hummus
- Added to soups for more protein
- Mixed with corn for a side salad

Recipes: *Vegetable and Black Bean Quesadillas, Grandma Lori's Baked Beans, White Bean Sandwich Spread*

• 5. BEETS •

Wonderful for eye health and full of fiber and potassium, beets benefit muscles, skin, and the neurological system. Their earthy flavor is an acquired taste for some, so get babies started on them early on. Roasting brings out their natural sweetness and makes a vibrant red mixture that kids get excited to dig into.

WAYS TO ENJOY

- Sliced thin and baked as chips
- Cooked and whirled into a smoothie
- Pickled (Really! Try it.)

Recipes: *Roasted Beets, Roasted Root Vegetables*

• 6. BELL PEPPERS •

It surprises parents to learn there is more vitamin C in a bell pepper than an orange. The sweet and juicy flavor makes them munchable on their own, plus they're great for dipping in homemade dips and salad dressings. Peppers also have high water content, so they help keep little bodies hydrated. The outer skin is a little tough, so raw peppers are best for kids with a full mouth of teeth.

WAYS TO ENJOY
- Sliced and dipped in homemade dressing or dip
- Stuffed with rice and ground turkey
- Diced and speckled on pizza

Recipes: *Vegetable and Black Bean Quesadillas, Veggie Kebabs, Three-Cheese Pizza, Veggie Scramble*

• 7. BERRIES •

Blueberries, raspberries, blackberries, strawberries, and cranberries are all filled with antioxidants called anthocyanins. They protect blood vessels and the nervous system and improve eyesight. Berries also offer vitamin C for skin health and vitamin K for healthy bones and circulation. Strawberries are considered a high-allergen food, so most pediatricians recommend waiting to introduce them until children are at least one year old.

WAYS TO ENJOY
- Drizzled with honey and a dollop of whipped cream
- Frozen in smoothies and frozen yogurt
- Added in or on top of pancakes and waffles

Recipes: *Cranberry-Lime Granita, Mixed Berry Pie Pockets, Fruit-Burst Ice Pops, Strawberry-Kiwi Fruit Leather, Grape Salsa, Blueberry–Greek Yogurt Mini Muffins, Nut-Free Granola, French Toast Sticks with Blackberry Sauce, Spoonable Smoothie, Yogurt Sundaes*

· 8. BISON ·

One of the leanest protein options around—low in fat but high in flavor. It's also an excellent source of minerals iron and zinc. Ground bison is the most readily available, and most large chain grocers carry it. You may be able to find steaks and tenderloin cuts at the farmers' market.

WAYS TO ENJOY
- Handmade burgers and meatballs
- Quick and easy taco night
- Mixed with marinara for meat sauce

Recipe: *Baked Bison Meatballs*

· 9. BROCCOLI ·

High in fiber and vitamins, broccoli boasts cell-protecting antioxidants plus a fun treelike shape that kids love to get their tiny hands on. The strong flavor might not appeal to small babies right away, but toddlers grow to love this nourishing superfood.

WAYS TO ENJOY
- Tossed broccoli salad: raw with raisins, cheese, and a little crispy bacon
- Roasted with olive oil, salt, and pepper
- Steamed with lemon and sea salt

Recipes: *Vegetable and Black Bean Quesadillas, Parmesan Roasted Broccoli with Brown Rice Pasta, Mac and Cheese with Vegetables and Chicken,*

Deconstructed Broccoli and Tofu Stir-Fry, Veggie Scramble

· 10. BROWN RICE ·

This whole grain packs in more tummy-pleasing fiber and protein plus ten times more energy-producing B vitamins (niacin, thiamin, and B6) compared to white rice. One half cup of cooked brown rice has 108 calories and a hefty dose of iron—4 percent of the daily recommendation for infants ages seven to twelve months and 6 percent for children ages one to three years. It also comes in many forms—brown rice crackers, breads, and pasta.

WAYS TO ENJOY
- Stir-fried with egg, soy sauce, and veggies
- Tossed with beans and fresh herbs
- Slow-cooked with milk and cinnamon

Recipes: *Parmesan Roasted Broccoli with Brown Rice Pasta, Brown Rice with Roasted Carrots, Cheesy Rice with Peas, Slow-Cooker Coconut Rice, Deconstructed Broccoli and Tofu Stir-Fry*

· 11. BUTTERNUT SQUASH ·

This winter squash is a true superfood. Loaded with vitamin A to benefit skin and vision, "BNS" (as we call it in my house) also contains vitamin C, energy boosting B vitamins, and heart-healthy potassium. It is absolutely delicious roasted with a little olive oil, salt, and pepper. One half cup of cooked squash has 40 calories and 1 gram of protein. Its bright orange color means it's bursting with beta-carotene—a cell-protecting anti-oxidant. This was a first veggie for both my girls, and they love it to this day.

WAYS TO ENJOY
- Roasted and mashed
- Pureed into sauce and soup
- Diced, boiled, and tossed with pasta and Parmesan

Recipes: *Butternut Squash Puree, Orange Crush, Charlie's Penne with Butternut Squash Sauce*

· 12. CARROTS ·

Carrots provide all kinds of nutrients important for growth and development, immunity, and vision. Babies as young as six months love the sweet flavor and soft texture of cooked carrots. Believe it or not, it is actually true that eating too many of these root veggies can turn a baby's skin orange! There is no need for alarm; it is completely harmless and will quickly resolve after a few days once fewer carrots are consumed.

WAYS TO ENJOY
- Juiced with fruits and veggies
- Shredded in cupcakes, muffins, and pancakes
- Sautéed with butter and fresh dill

Recipes: *Orange Crush, Carrot Marinara Sauce, Watermelon-Pineapple-Carrot Juice, Roasted Root*

Vegetables, Brown Rice with Roasted Carrots, Mac and Cheese with Vegetables and Chicken, Peanut Butter Spaghetti, Easy Chicken Soup, Slow-Cooker Lentil Soup, Egg Salad Sliders

· 13. CHEESE ·

Cheese has so much to offer growing bodies! It provides protein plus bone-building calcium, vitamin D, and phosphorus. Infants can typically start eating cheese around eight to nine months of age; mild flavors like Monterey Jack and American are typically tolerated best.

WAYS TO ENJOY
- Stirred up mac and cheese (cooked pasta, shredded cheddar, splash of milk)
- Baked mozzarella sticks (string cheese rolled in egg and panko)
- Sprinkled by tiny fingers on pizza and flatbread

Recipes: *Charlie's Penne with Butternut Squash Sauce; Vegetable and Black Bean Quesadillas; Parmesan Roasted Broccoli with Brown Rice Pasta; Zucchini Flatbread; Mac and Cheese with Vegetables and Chicken; Cheesy Rice with Peas; Three-Cheese Pizza; Whole Grain Chocolate Cupcakes with Cream Cheese and Mascarpone Frosting; Arugula Pesto Pasta; Buzz Burgers; Crispy Chicken Fingers with Magical Honey Mustard; Veggie Scramble; Lemon-Ricotta Cookies; Turkey and Cheese Panini; Paris-Inspired Omelet; Maddy's Special Egg Sandwich; Ham, Cheddar, and Basil Quiche Cups*

· 14. CHICKEN ·

Chicken provides lean protein for growing muscles. Its mild flavor makes it a good choice for infants just getting started with meats and other protein-rich solid foods. Contrary to popular belief, the majority of the fat in flavorful dark-meat chicken is the healthy, polyunsaturated kind.

WAYS TO ENJOY
- Soups and stocks
- Split bone-in breasts—roasted with olive oil, salt, and pepper
- Crispy baked chicken fingers

Recipes: *Mac and Cheese with Vegetables and Chicken, Easy Chicken Soup, Chicken Thighs with Sweet Potato, Crispy Chicken Fingers with Magical Honey Mustard*

· 15. COCOA ·

Yes, dark chocolate is a superfood thanks to the antioxidants, fiber, and iron found in cocoa powder. Chocolate does have the added sugar, of course, so give the kiddos dark chocolate in moderation.

WAYS TO ENJOY
- Homemade sauces and puddings
- Chocolate-dipped fruit
- Mini chips sprinkled over pancakes

Recipes: *Clementine Dippers, Whole Grain Chocolate Cupcakes with Cream Cheese and*

Mascarpone Frosting, Banana Chocolate Chip Bread, Chocolate-Dipped Pretzels, Nonni's Chocolate Pudding, Hot Chocolate

· 16. COCONUTS ·

An incredibly versatile fruit, rich and creamy coconut milk can be used as a cooking liquid for rice and noodle dishes. Boxed coconut milk (great for smoothies) is fortified with calcium and vitamin D, and nutrient-rich coconut water is a natural source of electrolytes (sodium and potassium). There are some questions as to whether those with tree nut allergies can eat coconuts (which are typically recognized as fruits), so check with an allergist if there are any questions.

WAYS TO ENJOY
- Toasted in granola
- Freeze coconut water into ice cubes and add to smoothies
- Pour coconut milk as cooking liquid for grains

Recipes: *Nut-Free Granola, Slow-Cooker Coconut Rice, Spoonable Smoothie*

· 17. CORN ·

Did you know corn is actually a whole grain? It is full of the antioxidant zeaxanthin, which benefits vision, plus it contains small amounts of protein and fiber. Whether you opt for popcorn or corn on the cob, corn helps to brighten up a dinner plate—kids just love it!

Popcorn can be a choking hazard, so save that for the kiddos ages two and up, but younger kids can happily chomp on fresh cobs and kernels.

WAYS TO ENJOY
- Mixed with peppers and tomatoes for corn salsa
- Added kernels to corn muffins
- Sprinkled with cheese and fresh herbs

Recipes: *Summer Squash "Pasta," Vegetable and Black Bean Quesadillas, Veggie Kebabs,* Real *Microwave Popcorn, Easy Chicken Soup*

· 18. CUCUMBER ·

Cukes make a fresh snack or a simple side salad. They are low in calories but high in water—veggies like this help keep little ones hydrated. We grow lots in our garden; the kids love to pick and eat them right there in the backyard. Peel off the skin for tiny ones, to prevent a choking hazard.

WAYS TO ENJOY
- Sliced and dunked into ice water
- Sliced and combined with soy sauce and sesame seeds
- Jarred homemade pickles

Recipes: *Cucumbers with Homemade Ranch Dressing, Peanut Butter Spaghetti*

· 19. EDAMAME ·

Soybeans are full of fiber, iron, and vitamins A and C. This plant-based source of protein makes an easy weeknight side dish. One-half cup has 88 calories and a whopping 10 grams of protein. Puree for babies, and let toddlers eat the whole beans as finger food.

WAYS TO ENJOY
- Steamed in the pods with salt
- Mashed into a sandwich spread
- Tossed in stir-fry

Recipe: *Whole Grain Pita Chips with Edamame Hummus*

· 20. EGGS ·

Egg whites and yolks are filled with protein. The yolk also contains vitamins A and D, as well as omega-3 fats for the brain, eyes, and skin. Egg whites carry a higher risk of allergic reaction, so introduce them separately from yolks to babies.

WAYS TO ENJOY
- Hard-boiled as a snack
- Baked quiche and frittata
- Scrambled breakfast burrito

35

Recipes: *Mixed Berry Pie Pockets; Whole Grain Pancakes; Blueberry–Greek Yogurt Mini Muffins; Whole Grain Chocolate Cupcakes with Cream Cheese and Mascarpone Frosting; Charlie's*

Double Pumpkin Muffins; French Toast Sticks with Blackberry Sauce; Baked Bison Meatballs; Panko-Breaded Fish Sticks; Veggie Scramble; Lemon-Ricotta Cookies; Paris-Inspired Omelet; Egg Salad Sliders; Maddy's Special Egg Sandwich; Ham, Cheddar, and Basil Quiche Cups

• 21. GRAPES •

Grapes hold lots of nutrients and antioxidants, plus a sweet and juicy burst that youngsters adore. Whole grapes are a choking hazard, so cut them up before serving. And don't count out dried grapes—naturally sweet raisins are a nutritious addition to muffins and oatmeal.

WAYS TO ENJOY
- Frozen and dunked in yogurt
- Threaded on skewers with grilled chicken
- Roasted and spooned into phyllo cups

Recipes: *Fruit-Burst Ice Pops, Grape Salsa, Cinnamon Roll Oatmeal*

• 22. GREEN BEANS •

36

Infants love this green veggie pureed, and toddlers love green beans for dipping. In addition to vitamins like K, C, and A, these beans also have about 1 milligram of iron per cup—that's more than 10 percent of the daily requirement for young children.

WAYS TO ENJOY

- Fresh from the garden
- Wrapped in bundles with bacon or ham
- Stir-fried with shrimp

Recipes: *Green Beans with Homemade French Dressing, Easy Chicken Soup*

· 23. HERBS ·

Fresh herbs add color, flavor, and nutrients to all kinds of recipes. Children love mild flavors like dill, parsley, thyme, and basil. Introduce foods flecked with green from the very beginning so kids grow into learning green foods are nothing to be afraid of.

WAYS TO ENJOY

- Pureed pesto—any herb will do
- Infused water
- Flavored marinades, soups, sauces, and dips

Recipes: *Smashed Potatoes with Fresh Dill; Cucumbers with Homemade Ranch Dressing; Easy Chicken Soup; Baked Bison Meatballs; Slow-Cooker Lentil Soup; White Bean Sandwich Spread; Paris-Inspired Omelet; Egg Salad Sliders; Ham, Cheddar, and Basil Quiche Cups*

· 24. HONEY ·

This natural sweetener contains minerals and antioxidants. Drizzle some on toast or oatmeal and use to sweeten up hummus and other dips. Honey should not be given to children less than one year old due to the risk of botulism.

WAYS TO ENJOY
- Honey-glazed vegetables
- Drizzled over muffins, waffles, and pancakes
- Naturally sweetened dipping sauces and salad dressings

Recipes: *Green Beans with Homemade French Dressing, Strawberry-Kiwi Fruit Leather, Dressed-Up Frozen Waffles with Pears and Honey, Whole Grain Pita Chips with Edamame Hummus, Banana Chocolate Chip Bread, Peanut Butter Spaghetti, Roasted Salmon, Crispy Chicken Fingers with Magical Honey Mustard, Yogurt Sundaes*

· 25. KALE ·

This newly popular green leafy vegetable can be turned into soup, salads, and even crunchy chips. Kale contains oodles of vitamin K, plus iron, potassium, calcium, and folate for healthy bones, muscles, and nerves. It can be a little bitter, so mix with mild fruits and veggies for babies and advance to plain as they grow.

WAYS TO ENJOY
- Blended into smoothies
- Finely chopped and sprinkled like parsley
- Wilted into soup

Recipes: *Green Machine, Kale Chips*

· 26. LENTILS ·

This nutritious legume is foreign to most families, but it's totally worth giving it a try! Kids love the soft chew and mild flavor of this high-protein powerhouse. Puree for babies between nine and twelve months of age.

WAYS TO ENJOY
- Homemade veggie burgers
- Tossed with rice
- Added to soup or salad to boost the protein

Recipe: *Slow-Cooker Lentil Soup*

· 27. MAPLE SYRUP ·

Along with honey, maple syrup is a wonderful option for a less processed sweetener. It still has the same calories as sugar, so make sure portions are modest. It is supersweet, so a little goes a long way. What kid doesn't love maple syrup on oatmeal, pancakes, and French toast?

WAYS TO ENJOY
- Mixed into oatmeal
- Drizzled on plain yogurt
- A less processed sweetener for baking

Recipes: *Whole Grain Pancakes, Blueberry–Greek Yogurt Mini Muffins, Nut-Free Granola, French Toast Sticks with Blackberry Sauce, Banana Chocolate Chip Bread, Grandma Lori's Baked Beans, Roasted Salmon, Yogurt Sundaes*

· 28. MELON ·

Whether it is cantaloupe, honeydew, or watermelon, you really can't go wrong. Fun colors and sweet flavors mean kids can't get enough. Antioxidants like beta-carotene and lycopene benefit cell health and eyesight.

WAYS TO ENJOY
- Juiced with lemon and apple
- Whirled into smoothies with berries and fresh lime
- Stacked melon balls as "snowmen"

Recipes: *Watermelon-Pineapple-Carrot Juice, Fruit-Burst Ice Pops, Grape Salsa, Yogurt Sundaes*

· 29. MILK ·

Milk is an excellent source of muscle and bone-building nutrients like protein, vitamin D, and calcium. Children can start drinking cow's milk after age one. Whole milk is typically the best choice because it provides the extra fat that a developing body needs. The switch can be made to lower fat milk (1 percent or 2 percent) once the child turns two. One cup of milk provides about 100 IU of vitamin D. Kids ages newborn to twelve months need 400 IU per day, while kids one to three years need 600. Milk is also rich in vitamin B12 and riboflavin for DNA formation and energy metabolism.

WAYS TO ENJOY
- Homemade flavored milk
- Heated cooking liquid for rice and oats
- Whipped-up milk shakes!

Recipes: *Maddy's Creamy Dreamy Banana Shake, Whole Grain Pancakes, Mac and Cheese with Vegetables and Chicken, Blueberry–Greek Yogurt Mini Muffins, Whole Grain Chocolate Cupcakes with Cream Cheese and Mascarpone Frosting, Breakfast Quinoa with Cherries, Charlie's Double Pumpkin Muffins, French Toast Sticks with Blackberry Sauce, Cinnamon Roll Oatmeal, Nonni's Chocolate Pudding, Lemon-Ricotta Cookies, Hot Chocolate*

· 30. OATS ·

This easy-to-cook whole grain contains vitamins, protein, and heart-healthy soluble fiber. Use it to make other kid favorites like granola and cookies. Puree and thin out with water, breast milk, or formula for babies.

WAYS TO ENJOY
- No-bake breakfast cookies with dried fruit, oats, and peanut butter
- Baked oatmeal chocolate chip cookies
- Added to pancake mix

Recipes: *Baby's First Oatmeal, Nut-Free Granola, Cinnamon Roll Oatmeal*

· 31. ORANGES (AND OTHER CITRUS) ·

Vitamin C is the obvious nutrient in this category, but there is also lots of hunger-fighting fiber. Little palates love the pucker-producing acidity from citrus fruits like oranges, grapefruit, lemons, and limes. Clementines are perfect for tiny hands; for a special treat, dip segments in dark chocolate.

WAYS TO ENJOY
- Squeezed OJ
- Simmered citrus marmalade
- Marinaded chicken and fish

Recipes: *Guac for All Ages, Quick Sautéed Peas, Peach Freezer Jam, Green Beans with Homemade French Dressing, Parmesan Roasted Broccoli with Brown Rice Pasta, Cranberry-Lime Granita, Mixed Berry Pie Pockets, Grape Salsa, Cucumbers with Homemade Ranch Dressing, Veggie Kebabs, Clementine Dippers, Blueberry–Greek Yogurt Mini Muffins, Cheesy Rice with Peas, French Toast Sticks with Blackberry Sauce, Arugula Pesto Pasta, Whole Grain Pita Chips with Edamame Hummus, Lemon Shrimp, Roasted Salmon, Peach-Swirl Yogurt, Lemon-Ricotta Cookies, White Bean Sandwich Spread, Tropical Milk Shake*

· 32. PASTA ·

Quite possibly every kid's favorite food, pasta is enriched with nutrients including B vitamins and iron. This carbohydrate-rich food is excellent fuel for active little ones. Whole grain versions should also be introduced early so children can acquire a taste for them, but start out with traditional pasta at about eight months of age because it is easier to digest.

WAYS TO ENJOY
- Cooked tortellini + salad dressing = pasta salad
- Twirled whole wheat pasta with garlic, lemon, and shrimp
- Baked in casseroles

Recipes: *Charlie's Penne with Butternut Squash Sauce, Parmesan Roasted Broccoli with Brown Rice Pasta, Mac and Cheese with Vegetables and Chicken, Arugula Pesto Pasta, Peanut Butter Spaghetti*

· 33. PEACHES ·

Peaches and other stone fruit like plums and apricots have fiber, vitamin C, and various antioxidants. Since they have such a short season, buy them at the farmers' market in the summer and frozen in the winter; they are just as healthy that way. Peeled, boiled, and pureed peaches make a velvety-smooth baby food for six- to eight-month-old babies.

WAYS TO ENJOY
- Chopped with cereal and milk
- Enjoyed solo as a snack
- Grilled with a little ice cream

43

Recipes: *Peach Freezer Jam, Peachy Parfaits, Peach-Swirl Yogurt, Spoonable Smoothie*

· 34. PEANUT BUTTER ·

This classic kid food is filled with heart-healthy fats, protein, fiber, and vitamin E. Peanuts also contain niacin, which is good for energy production. It is great for a good old PB&J or whisk into dips and sauces. Peanut butter does have a high allergy risk so hold off on giving it to kids until they are around the two-year mark. Ideally, look for a natural peanut butter with only peanuts and salt on the ingredient list. For those with food allergies, soy-nut butter and sunflower seed butter are tasty alternatives.

WAYS TO ENJOY
- Rolled-up PB&J pinwheels made with whole grain tortillas
- Stuffed in French toast
- Swirled into cooked oatmeal

Recipes: *Peanut Butter Spaghetti, Homemade Peanut Butter*

· 35. PEARS ·

A truly underappreciated fruit, pears are a serious source of fiber and vitamin K. Infants love the mildly sweet flavor when pureed. For older kids, tuck a pear in their lunch box or serve with cheese and crackers as an after-school snack.

WAYS TO ENJOY
- Simmer into pearsauce!

44

- Roasted and drizzled with honey
- Dried until supersweet and chewy

Recipes: *Dressed-Up Frozen Waffles with Pears and Honey, Yogurt Sundaes*

• 36. PEAS •

Kids love to munch on peas mixed with rice and pasta or solo as a side dish. Peas offer lots of protein and fiber, plus iron and zinc for healthy blood and immune system function. They puree beautifully for kids six to seven months old.

WAYS TO ENJOY
- Steamed, smashed, and spread on bread
- Added to pastas and soup to boost the protein and fiber
- Defrosted frozen peas + chicken broth + a blender = pea soup

Recipes: *Green Machine, Quick Sautéed Peas, Cheesy Rice with Peas, Easy Chicken Soup, Pork and Potatoes*

• 37. PINEAPPLE •

Pineapple offers plenty of vitamin C plus a mineral called manganese for healthy bones. Pineapple also contains an enzyme called bromelain, a potent anti-inflammatory.

- Mixed into yogurt and granola
- Dried as a sweet and chewy treat
- Frozen in a smoothie

Recipes: *Watermelon-Pineapple-Carrot Juice, Fruit-Burst Ice Pops, Grape Salsa, Spoonable Smoothie*

· 38. PORK ·

Cuts of pork like chops and tenderloin are high in protein and low in fat. They have more B vitamins than other types of meat. The mild flavor also appeals to many youngsters, so it's a good meat to serve to babies early on.

WAYS TO ENJOY
- Grilled and sliced for tacos and quesadillas
- Stir-fried pork fried rice
- Added to meatballs

Recipes: *Pork and Potatoes; Teriyaki Pork Tenderloin; Slow-Cooker Pulled Pork; Ham, Cheddar, and Basil Quiche Cups*

· 39. POTATOES ·

46

Potatoes contain fiber, protein, iron, and vitamin C (yes, there is vitamin C in potatoes). They are free of fat and cholesterol and contain more potassium than bananas, broccoli, and spinach. Enjoy pureed for infants or roasted as finger food for toddlers.

WAYS TO ENJOY

- Stuffed baked potatoes
- Sauteed potato pancakes
- Added to omelets and quiche

Recipes: *Smashed Potatoes with Fresh Dill, Crispy Oven Fries, Roasted Root Vegetables, Pork and Potatoes*

· 40. PUMPKIN ·

This underutilized squash makes a beautiful holiday pie but can also be used for soups, sauces, and puddings. It is high in vitamin A and antioxidants like beta-carotene and has a mild flavor that makes kids swoon. Puree for infants or roast and mash for older babies. Don't forget about the seeds—they're a tasty source of iron.

WAYS TO ENJOY

- Pureed and added to pancakes and French toast
- Pumpkin mousse = pumpkin puree folded into whipped cream
- Roasted pumpkin seeds

Recipe: *Charlie's Double Pumpkin Muffins*

· 41. QUINOA ·

This ingredient, pronounced *keen-wa*, can be cooked like oats or rice. It looks like a grain but is actually a seed, making it higher in protein. It is also gluten-free and high in iron, fiber, folate, and magnesium.

- Formed into quinoa burgers
- Mixed with black beans and veggies
- Cooked with broth or milk for extra flavor

Recipe: *Breakfast Quinoa with Cherries*

· 42. SEAFOOD ·
(Cod, Salmon, and Shrimp)

In June 2014, the FDA revised recommendations and increased the amount of fish that both pregnant women and children should be eating. Fish like cod, salmon, and shrimp are high in protein and a good source of omega-3 fats that are vital for brain development. They are low in mercury, a toxin that can have a negative effect on children and adults alike. Salmon contains vitamin D, which many youngsters are lacking. The mild flavor of cod makes it a perfect starter seafood for babies and toddlers. In general, fish is typically safe to introduce to babies between nine and twelve months, but hold off until two years for shellfish like shrimp and lobster, since they have a higher risk of allergic reaction.

WAYS TO ENJOY

- Canned salmon for burgers
- Poached or sautéed with fresh herbs
- Baked in parchment with fresh veggies

Recipes: *Panko-Breaded Fish Sticks, Lemon Shrimp, Roasted Salmon*

· 43. SPINACH ·

This powerful green veggie is filled with a long list of nutrients, including vitamins A, C, and K, plus minerals like iron, calcium, and zinc. Kids of all ages can enjoy; it is just as delicious as a puree as it is a pizza topper.

WAYS TO ENJOY
- Mixed into hot or cold spinach dip
- Wilted into pasta
- Steamed with fresh lemon

Recipes: *Spinach-Yogurt Puree, Green Machine, Vegetable and Black Bean Quesadillas, Veggie Scramble*

· 44. STOCKS ·

Whether it is chicken or vegetable, keep nutrient-rich stocks and broths on hand to make quick soups and sauces. Use in place of water to cook grains and add moisture to baby foods.

WAYS TO ENJOY
- Homemade soups
- Mixed with soy sauce and cornstarch to thicken stir-fry
- Cooked with grains, pasta, and risotto

49

Recipes: *Brown Rice with Roasted Carrots, Easy Chicken Soup, Slow-Cooker Lentil Soup*

· 45. SWEET POTATOES ·

This tuber lives up to its name—the natural sugars make it a favorite of tiny taste buds. Parents will be pleased to know sweet potatoes also boast plenty of fiber, vitamins, and antioxidants.

WAYS TO ENJOY
- Loaded sweet potato skins with cheese and broccoli
- Added to chili
- Baked, then mashed with butter and maple syrup

Recipes: *Orange Crush, Chicken Thighs with Sweet Potato*

· 46. TOFU ·

Don't be afraid of this high-protein meat alternative. With the proper preparation, everyone in the family will love it. Firm varieties are wonderful for roasting, while silken tofu makes a creamy smoothie. Tofu is also an excellent source of calcium.

WAYS TO ENJOY
- Sliced and roasted
- Blended for creamy smoothies
- Marinated and grilled

Recipes: *Deconstructed Broccoli and Tofu Stir-Fry*

· 47. TURKEY ·

This lean protein option is full of niacin, selenium, vitamin B6, phosphorus, and zinc, nutrients that assist with the health of bones, blood, and the immune system. From sandwiches to meatballs, turkey is a versatile ingredient for all kinds of kid-friendly foods.

WAYS TO ENJOY
- Ground for burgers and meatballs
- Roasted and sliced for sandwiches
- Boiled for stock

Recipes: *Buzz Burgers, Grilled Turkey Cutlets, Turkey and Cheese Panini*

· 48. WHOLE GRAIN BREADS AND FLOURS ·

Whether it is wheat, rye, oat, or multigrain, these breads contain more vitamins, minerals, protein, and fiber than processed white breads. Introducing these options to children from the very beginning will ensure better appreciation for the nutty flavor and better nutrition for a lifetime.

WAYS TO ENJOY
- Bread pudding
- Homemade bread crumbs and croutons
- Grilled cheese

Recipes: *Vegetable and Black Bean Quesadillas, Zucchini Flatbread, Whole Grain Pancakes,*

*Dressed-Up Frozen Waffles with Pears and Honey,
Blueberry–Greek Yogurt Mini Muffins, Three-
Cheese Pizza, Whole Grain Chocolate Cupcakes
with Cream Cheese and Mascarpone Frosting,
Charlie's Double Pumpkin Muffins, French Toast
Sticks with Blackberry Sauce, Whole Grain Pita
Chips with Edamame Hummus, Banana Chocolate
Chip Bread, Baked Bison Meatballs, Buzz Burgers,
Lemon-Ricotta Cookies, Turkey and Cheese Panini,
Egg Salad Sliders, Maddy's Special Egg Sandwich,
Yogurt Sundaes*

· 49. YOGURT ·

Yogurt is often the first dairy food recommended for
infants; they love the creamy texture and tangy flavor.
Yogurt also offers tummy-pleasing probiotics for digestion and intestinal health. With so many choices
for yogurt out there, parents are often left scratching
their heads in the dairy aisle. Fruit-flavored, whole milk
yogurt is a good place to start for infants. As they grow
older, start experimenting with lower fat options and
higher protein Greek varieties. One-half cup of plain,
low-fat yogurt has 71 calories and 6 grams of protein.
There is also a hefty dose of calcium and probiotics.
Many (but not all) yogurts are fortified with vitamin D;
check labels to make sure that the brand you feed your
little ones includes this important vitamin.

52

WAYS TO ENJOY
- Used to cut the fat in baking
- Whisked into dips
- Layered "sundaes" with fresh fruit and granola

Recipes: *Spinach-Yogurt Puree, Cucumbers with Homemade Ranch Dressing, Blueberry–Greek Yogurt Mini Muffins, Crispy Chicken Fingers with Magical Honey Mustard, Peach-Swirl Yogurt, Vanilla Bean Frozen Yogurt, Egg Salad Sliders, Yogurt Sundaes, Tropical Milk Shake*

· 50. ZUCCHINI ·

This low-calorie summer squash is always popular with infants and toddlers. It makes a light and flavorful puree for little ones. Shred and add to burgers or thinly slice for a pizza topping for toddlers.

WAYS TO ENJOY
- Shredded for muffins or pancakes
- Sliced and sautéed with oil and oregano
- Baked "Parmesan" style with cheese and sauce

Recipes: *Summer Squash "Pasta," Zucchini Flatbread, Veggie Kebabs*

· EQUIPPING YOUR KITCHEN ·

A few simple and affordable tools are all you need to make healthy and kid-friendly meals for children of all ages.

Ball Jars
An obvious choice for canning, you can use these decorative jars for storing homemade jams, pickles, salad dressings, sauces, and soups. They are dishwasher- and microwave-safe too. I prefer these to plastic, hands down!

Countertop Blender
A must-have for smoothies, shakes, and even juices. Waring and Vitamix are the best models you can buy, but there's no need to invest in a super-expensive machine.

Decent Knives
They don't have to be top of the line, but they do need to cut things without breaking your hand. Good knives are expensive, so be practical; a basic eight- to ten-inch chef's knife along with a good paring knife are a good place to start.

Food Mill
A food mill is by far the best tool for homemade baby food. Unplug and use this hand-cranked machine to make smooth purees as well as slightly chunky soups and sauces. OXO brand makes a sturdy food mill with three adjustable disks for different textures that will last for decades.

54

Food Processor

For everything from baby food to pesto to one-ingredient banana "ice cream," every kitchen should have a food processor. No need to go for the most expensive model; a standard seven- or nine-cup machine costs around $150.

Half Sheet Pans

A perfect-size pan for sweet and savory baking and roasting. Keep two or three of these 13 × 18 inch rectangular pans on hand for cookies, pizza, chicken, and fish. Most cooling racks and Silpats are made to fit these pans.

Ice-Cream Maker

This gadget is for so much more than ice cream; these handy machines are worth the reasonable investment for making tasty creations like frozen yogurt and fruit juice slushies. They do take up a fair amount of space, so plan ahead on a place to store it.

Immersion Blender

Lovingly called a "boat motor," immersion blenders can be placed directly into a large pot to instantly create smooth and velvety soups and sauces. It is not 100 percent necessary to have one if you have a countertop blender, but they are a huge time saver, especially on cleanup.

Julienne Peeler

A tiny handheld peeler that makes long and skinny strips of apples, carrots, cukes, potatoes, and summer squash for salads, sandwiches, pasta dishes, and soups. I use this tool at least once a day.

Mandoline Slicer

A magical tool for slicing all types of produce, a mandoline is especially helpful for harder, round items like beets and potatoes. For quick slicing of carrots, onions, and cucumbers, invest in a smaller handheld model; they are less cumbersome and easy to store.

Meat Thermometer

A cook's best tool for keeping food safe. Take the guesswork out of cooking meat by just checking the temperature. Parents can get more info from the Partnership for Food Safety Education. Their Fight Bac website (fightbac.org) helps teach kids (and parents) about food safety in the kitchen.

Parchment Paper

Nonstick paper that helps with everything from baking to keeping food fresh in freezer bags. Buy parchment in rolls or precut sheets that fit perfectly into half sheet pans.

Potato Masher

This low-tech kitchen tool is an obvious choice for mashed potatoes. It is also a secret weapon for guacamole.

Silpat Baking Mat

Silpat is a popular brand of nonstick baking mat for cookies, pastries, candies, and other sticky concoctions. If you bake a lot you need one of these.

3

~~~~~~

Fruit and Vegetable
Recipes

· 6 TO 12 MONTHS ·

Basic Fruit and Veggie Purees

Making from-scratch baby food is so much easier than most people think. Once you start, you'll be hooked. You can find some good brands of jarred foods out there nowadays, but I've never had to buy one with these recipes on hand!

Ingredients: fresh or frozen fruits and vegetables, chopped and peels removed where applicable. Just about all of the superfoods can be made into purees of some sort—let your creativity run wild.

Method 1

Place food in a medium saucepan and cover with water. Bring mixture to a boil, reduce heat, and simmer until tender. Drain, reserving some of the cooking liquid. Puree with a blender, food processor, or food mill and thin out with reserved cooking liquid as needed.

Method 2

Roast on a baking sheet at 400°F until tender. Puree with a blender, food processor, or food mill and thin with water as needed.

Storage: Store purees in the refrigerator for up to five days. Freeze in small batches for up to three months. Place in ice cube trays and, once frozen, pop out and place in a freezer-safe bag. Defrost in a saucepan on the stovetop or in the microwave.

Perfect Applesauce

Most of the time, simple is best! This recipe is a favorite for kids of all ages. As children grow older, modify this recipe by adding cinnamon or even strawberries to the mix.

4 pounds **apples**, peeled, cored, and diced

½ cup water

Combine ingredients in a large pot and cook over medium heat until apples are tender, 20 to 30 minutes. Pass through a food mill to reach desired consistency. For baby's first food, use the finest setting.

▶ **YIELD:** 1 quart

Nutrition Information per ¼ Cup
Calories: 48, Total Fat: 0 grams, Saturated Fat: 0 grams, Carbohydrate: 13 grams, Sugars: 10 grams, Protein: 0 grams, Sodium: 0 milligrams, Cholesterol: 0 milligrams, Fiber: 1 gram, Vitamin D: 0 IU, Calcium: 5 milligrams, Iron: 0 milligrams

Butternut Squash Puree

This velvety-smooth puree is a perfect first veggie for infants discovering solid foods. As little ones grow, you can use this recipe to make soups and pasta sauces by adding a few simple ingredients. In this recipe, the use of the cooking liquid helps retain nutrients.

1 medium **butternut squash** (2 pounds), peeled, seeded, and diced

Place diced squash in a large pot and cover with water. Bring to a boil, reduce to a simmer, and cook until squash is tender, about 15 minutes. Drain, reserving 1 cup of the cooking liquid. Place cooked squash in a blender along with ½ cup of the cooking liquid and puree. Thin out more with additional cooking liquid if desired.

▶ **YIELD:** 2½ cups

Nutrition Information per ¼ Cup
Calories: 31, Total Fat: 0 grams, Saturated Fat: 0 grams, Carbohydrate: 8 grams, Sugars: 2 grams, Protein: 1 gram, Sodium: 4 milligrams, Cholesterol: 0 milligrams, Fiber: 1 gram, Vitamin D: 0 IU, Calcium: 25 milligrams, Iron: 0.5 milligrams

Guac for All Ages

~~~~~~~~~

Avocados are a beautiful early food to introduce to tiny palates because they just love the creamy texture. This fruit (yes, it's technically a fruit) is loaded with vitamins, antioxidants, and healthy fats. Warning: Avocado gets messy—but it's OK—it's all part of the fun of learning how to eat.

2 ripe **avocados**
Juice of ½ a **lime***
Pinch of kosher salt*

Cut the avocados in half, remove the pit, and scoop out the flesh into a medium bowl. Pass through a food mill or mash well with a fork or potato masher. Thin out with a little water if needed.

* Serve plain to babies ages four to six months; mix with lime juice and salt for older children.

▶ **YIELD:** 1 cup

Nutrition Information per 1 Tablespoon
Calories: 24, Total Fat: 2 grams, Saturated Fat: 0 grams, Carbohydrate: 1 gram, Sugars: 0 grams, Protein: 0 grams, Sodium: 10 milligrams, Cholesterol: 0 milligrams, Fiber: 1 gram, Vitamin D: 0 IU, Calcium: 2 milligrams, Iron: 0 milligrams

Spinach-Yogurt Puree

~~~~~~~~~~

Spinach is an iron-rich leafy green veggie. Despite its slightly bitter flavor, many babies love it! Around eight months of age, yogurt can be introduced into the diet. Once your baby has tried yogurt solo, combine with fruits and veggies for a deliciously healthy and more satisfying meal. No need for picking through a large bag of fresh greens; a bag of frozen spinach works perfectly for this recipe.

1 (16-ounce) bag frozen, cut leaf **spinach**
¼ cup plain whole milk **yogurt**

Thaw spinach in the microwave (check bag for directions), cool slightly, and squeeze out any excess liquid. Place spinach in a food processor or blender and blend until smooth. Add yogurt and pulse until well combined.

▶ **YIELD:** about 3 cups

Nutrition Information per ¼ Cup
Calories: 12, Total Fat: 0 grams, Saturated Fat: 0 grams, Carbohydrate: 2 grams, Sugars: 0 grams, Protein: 1 gram, Sodium: 60 milligrams, Cholesterol: 1 milligram, Fiber: 1 gram, Vitamin D: 0.1 IU, Calcium: 42 milligrams, Iron: 0.6 milligrams

Roasted Bananas with Cinnamon

~~~~~~~~~~

The warmth of the oven brings out the natural sweetness of bananas, and the kitchen will be filled with the aroma of cinnamon. Freeze leftovers and blend with milk for an amazingly delicious smoothie.

1 medium **banana**
⅛ teaspoon ground cinnamon

Preheat oven to 400°F. Leaving the peel on, split the banana lengthwise and place on a baking sheet. Sprinkle with cinnamon and roast for 15 to 20 minutes or until warm. Scoop out, mash to desired consistency, and serve.

▶ **YIELD:** 1 banana

Nutrition Information per ½ Banana
Calories: 53 , Total Fat: 0 grams, Saturated Fat: 0 grams, Carbohydrate: 14 grams, Sugars: 7 grams, Protein: 1 gram, Sodium: 1 milligram, Cholesterol: 0 milligrams, Fiber: 2 grams, Vitamin D: 0 IU, Calcium: 4 milligrams, Iron: 0.2 milligrams

Orange Crush

~~~~~~~~~~

Babies will gobble up every last bit of this naturally sweet vegetable trio. Chop all the veggies approximately the same size for even cooking. When babies get older, puree in some cooked chicken.

2 **carrots**, peeled and chopped (about 1 cup)

1 small **sweet potato**, peeled and chopped (about 1 cup)

1 cup diced **butternut squash**

Place all ingredients in a small saucepan and cover with water. Bring to a boil and reduce heat to medium. Cook for 15 to 20 minutes or until vegetables are fork-tender. Drain, reserving the cooking liquid. Transfer the cooked vegetables to a food processor and blend until smooth. Add the cooking liquid in small amounts until mixture reaches desired consistency.

▶ **YIELD:** 1 cup

Nutrition Information per ¼ Cup
Calories: 19, Total Fat: 0 grams, Saturated Fat: 0 grams, Carbohydrate: 5 grams, Sugars: 1 gram, Protein: 0 grams, Sodium: 14 milligrams, Cholesterol: 0 milligrams, Fiber: 1 gram, Vitamin D: 0 IU, Calcium: 12 milligrams, Iron: 0.2 milligrams

Green Machine

~~~~~~~~~~

There's no denying the nutrition found in these three green vegetables. Get little ones started on these super-foods right from the beginning. Add Parmesan cheese and toss with pasta for older children.

2 cups chopped fresh **kale**
1 cup frozen **peas**
1 cup thawed frozen **spinach**

Place all ingredients in a small saucepan and cover with water. Bring to a boil and reduce heat to medium. Cook for 5 minutes. Drain, reserving the cooking liquid. Transfer the cooked vegetables to a food processor and blend until smooth; add the cooking liquid in small amounts until mixture reaches desired consistency.

▶ **YIELD:** about 3 cups

Nutrition Information per ¼ Cup
Calories: 18, Total Fat: 0 grams, Saturated Fat: 0 grams, Carbohydrate: 3 grams, Sugars: 1 gram, Protein: 1 gram, Sodium: 16 milligrams, Cholesterol: 0 milligrams, Fiber: 1 gram, Vitamin D: 0 IU, Calcium: 32 milligrams, Iron: 0.5 milligrams

Banana "Ice Cream"

"Ice cream" that even the youngest of babies can enjoy. This frozen treat is a delightful option for sore gums or a boo-boo on the mouth. As children grow, mix in their favorite toppings.

4 **bananas**, chopped and frozen

Place bananas in food processor and pulse until smooth and creamy.

▶ **YIELD:** 2 cups

Nutrition Information per ¼ Cup
Calories: 53, Total Fat: 0 grams, Saturated Fat: 0 grams, Carbohydrate: 13 grams, Sugars: 7 grams, Protein: 1 gram, Sodium: 1 milligram, Cholesterol: 0 milligrams, Fiber: 2 grams, Vitamin D: 0 IU, Calcium: 3 milligrams, Iron: 0.2 milligrams

Charlie's Penne with Butternut Squash Sauce

Take a break from marinara with this nutrient-filled sauce. Butternut squash gives it subtle sweetness and a gorgeous orange hue. This pasta dish has the essence of mac and cheese with much less fat.

8 ounces penne **pasta**

2 tablespoons heavy cream

1 cup Butternut Squash Puree (page 60)

2 tablespoons grated **Parmesan cheese**

Cook pasta according to package directions. Drain and set aside. In the same pot heat the cream until it comes to a simmer. Add butternut squash puree, stir until well combined. Add pasta and cheese, toss well, and serve.

▶ **YIELD:** 4 cups

Nutrition Information per ½ Cup
Calories: 138, Total Fat: 2 grams, Saturated Fat: 1 gram, Carbohydrate: 24 grams, Sugars: 1 gram, Protein: 5 grams, Sodium: 34 milligrams, Cholesterol: 7 milligrams, Fiber: 1 gram, Vitamin D: 1 IU, Calcium: 40 milligrams, Iron: 1 milligram

Carrot Marinara Sauce

I'm not a big fan of sneaking veggies into my kids' meals, but I love that marinara sauce is a blended-up version of all kinds of healthy produce. I often have left-over cooked carrots in the fridge, and since I hate to waste anything, this sauce was created. Use carrots that have been roasted, steamed, or frozen and thawed. Try with other veggies or make with just tomatoes—this is my basic no-fail tomato sauce recipe for pizza and pasta.

2 tablespoons extra virgin olive oil

1 clove garlic, chopped

½ medium onion, chopped

½ teaspoon ground fennel seed

1 (28-ounce) can crushed tomatoes

1 cup cooked **carrots**

1 teaspoon granulated sugar

Kosher salt and black pepper

1 cup fresh **basil** leaves

Heat oil in a medium saucepan. Add garlic and onion and sauté for 5 minutes. Add ground fennel and cook for 20 seconds, until fragrant. Add tomatoes, carrots, and sugar; season with ½ teaspoon salt and black pepper to taste. Cook, uncovered, for 20 minutes, stirring occasionally. Add basil and season with additional salt and pepper, if needed. Puree sauce using an immersion blender until smooth.*

* If you do not have an immersion blender, puree in a countertop blender in small batches. Make sure to hold the top of the blender closed with a dish towel while the machine is on.

▶ **YIELD:** 1 quart

Nutrition Information per ¼ Cup
Calories: 37, Total Fat: 2 grams, Saturated Fat: 0.5 grams, Carbohydrate: 5 grams, Sugars: 1 gram, Protein: 1 gram, Sodium: 105 milligrams, Cholesterol: 0 milligrams, Fiber: 1 gram, Vitamin D: 0 IU, Calcium: 25 milligrams, Iron: 0.8 milligrams

Quick Sautéed Peas

~~~~~~~~~

Instead of tossing peas in the microwave, make them a little more special. Frozen peas work perfectly for this recipe—no need to thaw! Puree with some chicken stock, and you have a fresh and fast pea soup.

2 teaspoons olive oil
2 cups frozen **peas**
Juice of ½ a **lemon**
Sea salt or kosher salt

Heat oil in a medium skillet over medium-high heat. Add peas and lemon; season with salt to taste and cook for 3 to 4 minutes until warmed through.

▶ **YIELD:** 2 cups

Nutrition Information per ¼ Cup
Calories: 7, Total Fat: 0 grams, Saturated Fat: 0 grams, Carbohydrate: 1 gram, Sugars: 1 gram, Protein: 1 gram, Sodium: 36 milligrams, Cholesterol: 0 milligrams, Fiber: 0.5 grams, Vitamin D: 0 IU, Calcium: 7 milligrams, Iron: 0.3 milligrams

Roasted Beets

Believe it or not, kids love *beets! The sooner you get them hooked, the better. Tiny roasted pieces make bright red finger food for toddlers, or puree into a velvety-smooth mixture for babies. If you pick beets up at the farmers' market, don't waste the delicious and nutritious greens; they can be used just like spinach.*

2 cups diced **beets** (about 3 medium beets)
1 tablespoon olive oil
½ teaspoon kosher salt

Preheat oven to 400°F. Place beets on a sheet pan, drizzle with olive oil and salt, and toss well to coat. Roast for 15 to 20 minutes or until pieces are fork-tender. Puree with a blender, food processor, or food mill. Thin with water as needed.

▶ **YIELD:** 2 cups

Nutrition Information per ¼ Cup
Calories: 30, Total Fat: 2 grams, Saturated Fat: 0 grams, Carbohydrate: 3 grams, Sugars: 2 grams, Protein: 1 gram, Sodium: 97 milligrams, Cholesterol: 0 milligrams, Fiber: 1 gram, Vitamin D: 0 IU, Calcium: 5 milligrams, Iron: 0.3 milligrams

Summer Squash "Pasta"

Later in the summer I'm always looking for something new to do with the zucchini I have all over the kitchen counter. The whole house complains ("Zucchini again?!"), but they don't mean it. This dish is all about the flavors from the family garden. A Zyliss julienne peeler is my tool of choice for making easy strips of squash.

3 large **zucchini**, unpeeled

1 tablespoon olive oil

1 cup cherry tomatoes, halved

1 cup **corn** kernels (preferably fresh but can be frozen)

¾ teaspoon kosher salt

1 teaspoon chopped fresh **oregano**

Using a vegetable peeler, strip zucchini into thin ribbons. Heat oil in a large skillet over medium heat. Add zucchini, tomatoes, and corn; season with salt and oregano and cook until vegetables are slightly wilted and warm, about 5 minutes.

▶ **YIELD:** about 5 cups

Nutrition Information per ½ Cup
Calories: 44, Total Fat: 2 grams, Saturated Fat: 0 grams, Carbohydrate: 6 grams, Sugars: 4 grams, Protein: 2 grams, Sodium: 75 milligrams, Cholesterol: 0 milligrams, Fiber: 1 gram, Vitamin D: 0 IU, Calcium: 19 milligrams, Iron: 0.5 milligrams

Peach Freezer Jam

~~~~~~~

I love the quality and flavor of homemade jam—it's a tremendous way to hold on to the flavors of summer—but I don't always have time for the traditional canning process. Freezer jam solved that problem! Look for no-sugar-needed pectin in the grocery store specialty aisle during the summer months or buy it online year-round. Use this same method for other fruits like berries, plums, and apricots.

2 cups granulated sugar

3 tablespoons no-sugar-needed pectin

4 cups peeled and chopped **peaches**

Juice of 1 **lemon**

Stir together sugar and pectin in bowl and set aside. In a large saucepan combine fruit and lemon juice. Bring mixture to a simmer over medium-high heat. Stir in sugar and pectin mixture and bring to a hard boil. Boil for 1 minute, remove from heat. Ladle jam into freezer-safe containers, cover, and place aside to set for 2 hours. Transfer to freezer and store for up to 6 months. When ready to use, transfer to the fridge for up to 1 month.

▶ **YIELD:** 3 cups

Nutrition Information per Tablespoon
Calories: 40, Total Fat: 0 grams, Saturated Fat: 0 grams, Carbohydrate: 10 grams, Sugars: 10 grams, Protein: 0 grams, Sodium: 0 milligrams, Cholesterol: 0 milligrams, Fiber: 0 grams, Vitamin D: 0 IU, Calcium: 2 milligrams, Iron: 0 milligrams

Maddy's Creamy Dreamy Banana Shake

〜〜〜〜〜〜

My older daughter can't get enough of this "milk shake," where frozen banana takes the place of ice cream. To turn into a breakfast item, add a handful of fresh berries, or throw in some mini chocolate chips and—voilà—it's dessert.

2 medium **bananas**, frozen

1 cup low-fat (1 percent) **milk**

Place ingredients in a blender and blend until smooth.

▶ **YIELD:** about 2½ cups

Nutrition Information per ½ Cup
Calories: 102, Total Fat: 1 gram, Saturated Fat: 1 gram, Carbohydrate: 22 grams, Sugars: 14 grams, Protein: 4 grams, Sodium: 42 milligrams, Cholesterol: 5 milligrams, Fiber: 2 grams, Vitamin D: 33 IU, Calcium: 104 milligrams, Iron: 0.2 milligrams

Watermelon-Pineapple-Carrot Juice

~~~~~~~~~

Nowadays juicing is trendy for everyone, even kids! But don't believe all the hype. Juices are tasty for an occasional thirst quencher, but juicing destroys some nutrients and should not be a full-time replacement for whole fruits and veggies. No juicer? No problem! Make this gorgeous and delicious sipper with a blender and a fine mesh strainer.

1 cup chopped fresh **watermelon**

1 cup chopped fresh **pineapple**

1 large **carrot**, chopped

¼ cup water

Run ingredients through a juicer or place in a blender and blend until smooth. Pour mixture through a fine mesh strainer to remove pulp if desired. Transfer to a container and shake well before serving.

▶ **YIELD:** 1½ cups (about 1 cup if strained)

Nutrition Information per ½ Cup
Calories: 53, Total Fat: 0 grams, Saturated Fat: 0 grams, Carbohydrate: 13 grams, Sugars: 10 grams, Protein: 1 gram, Sodium: 18 milligrams, Cholesterol: 0 milligrams, Fiber: 2 grams, Vitamin D: 0 IU, Calcium: 20 milligrams, Iron: 0.4 milligrams

Green Beans with Homemade French Dressing

~~~~~~~

Tangy French dressing brings back fuzzy childhood memories of Day-Glo bottled dressing, but now I know better. Store-bought versions of most salad dressings are loaded with sugar, preservatives, and artificial colors. This recipe has all the flavor but none of the junk. It makes a terrific dipping sauce for vegetables, chicken, or shrimp.

1 tablespoon white vinegar

Juice of ½ a **lemon**

1 tablespoon **honey**

¼ cup ketchup

1 teaspoon mustard powder

1 teaspoon paprika

½ teaspoon kosher salt

⅓ cup olive oil

1 pound **green beans**, trimmed and steamed

In a blender, combine vinegar, lemon juice, honey, ketchup, mustard powder, paprika, and salt. With the machine running, slowly pour in olive oil until all is incorporated and dressing is thickened. Serve with steamed green beans.

▶ **YIELD:** ½ cup dressing

Nutrition Information per Serving
(½ Cup Green Beans and 1 Tablespoon Dressing)
Calories: 119, Total Fat: 9 grams, Saturated Fat: 1 gram, Carbohydrate: 9 grams, Sugars: 5 grams, Protein: 1 gram, Sodium: 155 milligrams, Cholesterol: 0 milligrams, Fiber: 2 grams, Vitamin D: 0 IU, Calcium: 30 milligrams, Iron: 0.5 milligrams

Vegetable and Black Bean Quesadillas

~~~~~~~~~~

This is a go-to meal for Meatless Monday dinners, weekend lunches, or any other day when my kids decide they suddenly don't like meat. There's plenty of healthy plant-based protein in this easy-to-prepare recipe.

2 ounces shredded or sliced **cheese**

1 (6-inch) **whole wheat flour tortilla**

¼ cup canned **black beans**, rinsed and drained

½ cup cooked or raw vegetables (such as **bell peppers**, **broccoli**, **corn**, and **spinach**)

Place half of the cheese on half of the tortilla, followed by beans, vegetables, and remaining cheese. Fold in half and cook in a nonstick skillet for 3 minutes per side or microwave for 30 seconds per side on high. Allow to cool slightly before slicing into four wedges.

▶ **YIELD:** 1 quesadilla

Nutrition Information per ¼ Quesadilla
Calories: 102, Total Fat: 5 grams, Saturated Fat: 3 grams, Carbohydrate: 8 grams, Sugars: 0 grams, Protein: 6 grams, Sodium: 144 milligrams, Cholesterol: 15 milligrams, Fiber: 2 grams, Vitamin D: 4 IU, Calcium: 123 milligrams, Iron: 0.7 milligrams

Parmesan Roasted Broccoli with Brown Rice Pasta

~~~~~~~~

Brown rice pasta is a useful option for households where kids would be perfectly content eating pasta seven nights a week. It's also a whole grain and gluten-free option for families with allergies. Nowadays you can find it at most grocery stores, but some brands are better than others—I like Trader Joe's and Tinkyada. Serve this dish with roasted chicken or grilled shrimp, or toss in some white beans for a Meatless Monday dinner.

12 ounces **brown rice** pasta

3 cups **broccoli** florets, cut into bite-size pieces

2 tablespoons olive oil, divided

½ teaspoon kosher salt

2 tablespoons grated **Parmesan cheese**

Zest and juice of ½ a **lemon**

Cook pasta according to package directions and set aside. Preheat oven to 400°F. Place broccoli on a sheet pan, drizzle with 1 tablespoon olive oil, and season with salt. Roast for 10 to 12 minutes or until crisp-tender. Remove from oven and toss with Parmesan, lemon zest, and lemon juice. Toss broccoli with cooked pasta and serve.

▶ **YIELD:** 7 cups

Nutrition Information per 1 Cup
Calories: 227, Total Fat: 6 grams, Saturated Fat: 1 gram, Carbohydrate: 40 grams, Sugars: 1 gram, Protein: 5 grams, Sodium: 117 milligrams, Cholesterol: 1 milligram, Fiber: 3 grams, Vitamin D: 0 IU, Calcium: 38 milligrams, Iron: 0.4 milligrams

Smashed Potatoes with Fresh Dill

Need a healthy and delish side dish on the table fast? These quick-cooking potatoes are ready in 20 minutes. Kids love to help with the smashing. If seeing green specks in their food tends to freak out your kids, get them involved in the cooking; it will show them that the dill is nothing to be afraid of.

1 pound small red **potatoes**

2 tablespoons butter or buttery spread such as Smart Balance

½ teaspoon kosher salt

¼ teaspoon black pepper

¼ cup fresh chopped **dill**

Place potatoes in a medium saucepan and cover with cold water. Bring to a boil, reduce to a simmer, and cook for approximately 20 minutes, until potatoes are fork-tender. Drain and return to pot. Add butter, salt, pepper, and dill and smash with a fork or potato masher.

▶ **YIELD:** about 2½ cups

Nutrition Information per ¼ Cup
Calories: 34, Total Fat: 2 grams, Saturated Fat: 1 gram, Carbohydrate: 3 grams, Sugars: 0 grams, Protein: 0 grams, Sodium: 57 milligrams, Cholesterol: 6 milligrams, Fiber: 0 grams, Vitamin D: 2 IU, Calcium: 3 milligrams, Iron: 0.2 milligrams

Kale Chips

~~~~~~~~~~~~

Kale chips are a colorful alternative to greasy chips. Everyone can benefit from eating more kale, and these crispy chips help make it deliciously easy. You can now find these packaged in the chip section of most grocery stores, but making your own is much more cost-effective. Add flavor with a pinch of ground spices like cumin, paprika, or mild curry powder.

1 large bunch **kale**, stems removed and roughly chopped (6 to 8 cups)

2 tablespoons olive oil

Kosher salt and black pepper

Preheat oven to 400°F. Place kale on baking sheet. Drizzle with oil, sprinkle with salt and pepper to taste, and toss well. Bake for 3 to 5 minutes, turning once or until leaves just become crispy.

▶ **YIELD:** 6 to 8 cups

Nutrition Information per ½ Cup
Calories: 24, Total Fat: 1 gram, Saturated Fat: 0 grams, Carbohydrate: 3 grams, Sugars: 0 grams, Protein: 1 gram, Sodium: 32 milligrams, Cholesterol: 0 milligrams, Fiber: 1 gram, Vitamin D: 0 IU, Calcium: 45 milligrams, Iron: 0.6 milligrams

Crispy Oven Fries

Potatoes are loaded with potassium, fiber, and iron. These golden and crispy fries are a staple in my house—you'll never miss the deep-fried version.

4 large Yukon gold **potatoes**, scrubbed*
2 tablespoons olive oil
Sea salt and black pepper to taste

Preheat oven to 400°F. Cut potatoes into evenly sized strips. Place on a baking sheet, drizzle with olive oil, and season with salt and pepper. Bake for 35 to 40 minutes, tossing frequently, until crisp and golden.

* Peel for younger children to prevent choking.

▶ **YIELD:** 8 servings

Nutrition Information per Serving
Calories: 112, Total Fat: 3 grams, Saturated Fat: 0 grams, Carbohydrate: 19 grams, Sugars: 1 gram, Protein: 2 grams, Sodium: 76 milligrams, Cholesterol: 0 milligrams, Fiber: 2 grams, Vitamin D: 0 IU, Calcium: 13 milligrams, Iron: 0.9 milligrams

Mixed Berry Pie Pockets

Baking is not my strong suit, especially when it comes to pies and pastries. I keep working at it, but on most days instead of fumbling with pastry dough, I'd rather take the kids to the local farmers' market while prepared puff pastry defrosts in the fridge. When we get home we make these delectable handheld treats.

1 **egg**

1 tablespoon water

½ cup fresh or frozen mixed **berries***

1 tablespoon granulated sugar

1 teaspoon cornstarch

Juice of ½ a **lemon**

1 (14 × 9 inch) sheet trans-fat-free puff pastry (Dufour brand recommended)

Sparkling sugar (optional)

Line a baking sheet with parchment or a Silpat baking mat, set aside. Preheat oven to 400°F. Combine egg and water in a small bowl, beat well, and set aside.

In a medium bowl, combine berries, sugar, cornstarch, and lemon juice; stir to combine, then set aside.

Turn out puff pastry onto a lightly floured surface, roll out gently to flatten, but be careful not to press down too hard. Use a paring knife or pizza cutter to cut pastry in half, then cut each half into four rectangles so you are left with eight evenly sized pieces. Place one heaping tablespoon of the berry mixture in the center of each piece of pastry. Brush one side with egg wash; fold in half to form a square. Seal the edges with your fingers or a fork and transfer to prepared baking sheet.

Using a paring knife, cut a small slit in each piece. Brush the tops with egg wash and sprinkle with sparkling sugar, if desired. Bake for 10 to 12 minutes, until golden. Allow to cool on the sheet for at least 15 minutes before serving.

* If using frozen fruit, combine ingredients in a small saucepan and heat until all ingredients are well combined; allow to cool completely before continuing.

▶ **YIELD:** 8 pieces

Nutrition Information per Piece
Calories: 220, Total Fat: 16 grams, Saturated Fat: 10 grams, Carbohydrate: 16 grams, Sugars: 2 grams, Protein: 2 grams, Sodium: 165 milligrams, Cholesterol: 43 milligrams, Fiber: 0 grams, Vitamin D: 0 IU, Calcium: 1 milligram, Iron: 0 milligrams

Cranberry-Lime Granita

~~~~~~~~~~~

This is my less processed answer to snow cones and Italian ice. This refreshing and crunchy spoonable mixture is the ultimate summertime treat. Get the kids in the kitchen to help with the scraping. Make it extra special with a dollop of freshly whipped cream.

3½ cups **cranberry** juice cocktail
½ cup freshly squeezed **lime** juice
½ cup granulated sugar

Combine cranberry juice, lime juice, and sugar into a large saucepan. Heat over medium heat for 2 to 3 minutes, until sugar is dissolved. Transfer to a shallow glass container (such as a 9 × 13 × 2 inch baking dish); allow to cool slightly, then place in the freezer. Once the mixture begins to freeze, scrape with a fork every 30 minutes to create ice crystals until mixture is completely frozen. To serve, spoon into cups.

▶ **YIELD:** about 4 cups

Nutrition Information per ½ Cup
Calories: 113, Total Fat: 0 grams, Saturated Fat: 0 grams, Carbohydrate: 29 grams, Sugars: 27 grams, Protein: 0 grams, Sodium: 7 milligrams, Cholesterol: 0 milligrams, Fiber: 0 grams, Vitamin D: 0 IU, Calcium: 43 milligrams, Iron: 0 milligrams

84

Strawberry-Kiwi Fruit Leather

Commercially prepared fruit leathers are filled with highly processed sweeteners and even trans fats! This recipe is made from whole-food ingredients and keeps the sugar content in check. Take the kids berry picking and hold on to the tasty memories a bit longer. It is just as easy to double or triple this recipe, but be sure to use separate sheet pans for each batch to get the proper thickness and cooking time. This recipe is a little time-consuming but most of the time is inactive. The hardest part will be waiting to dig in.

1½ cups chopped fresh **strawberries**

½ cup chopped fresh kiwi

2 tablespoons **honey**

2 tablespoons sugar

Preheat oven to 170°F. Line a baking sheet with parchment paper or a Silpat mat and set aside. Place fruit, honey, and sugar in a medium saucepan. Bring to a boil and cook for about 5 minutes, then puree using an immersion blender.* Continue to cook over medium-high heat for an additional 10 to 15 minutes or until thick and syrupy; the mixture should be thick enough to coat the back of a spoon. Pour the hot fruit mixture onto prepared baking sheet and spread evenly into approximately an 8 × 12 inch rectangle. Place in the oven and bake for 3 hours. After 3 hours have passed, turn off the oven and allow to sit overnight. Cut into strips with a pizza cutter; roll up in a clean piece of parchment paper. Store in an airtight container for up to 3 weeks.

* If you do not have an immersion blender, puree in a food processor and then return mixture to saucepan.

▶ **YIELD:** 12 strips

Nutrition Information per 1 Strip
Calories: 21, Total Fat: 0 grams, Saturated Fat: 0 grams, Carbohydrate: 5 grams, Sugars: 4 grams, Protein: 0 grams, Sodium: 1 milligram, Cholesterol: 0 milligrams, Fiber: 1 gram, Vitamin D: 0 IU, Calcium: 6 milligrams, Iron: 0.1 milligrams

Fruit-Burst Ice Pops

These popsicles are made with 100 percent real fruit—you won't find that in the freezer aisle. They work wonders on sore gums when teething or on a hot day playing in the backyard. Experiment with different kinds of juice; just make sure they're all 100 percent fruit juice, made without added sugars.

1 cup 100 percent white **grape** juice

1 cup water

Finely chopped fresh fruit (**berries**, **grapes**, **pineapple**, **cantaloupe**)

Combine juice and water in a large measuring cup; stir to combine. Pour juice into ice pop molds, filling about three-quarters of the way full. Drop in pieces of fresh fruit and insert sticks and caps as directed. Transfer to the freezer for at least 4 hours to harden.

▶ **YIELD:** 6 ice pops

Nutrition Information per Pop
Calories: 38, Total Fat: 0 grams, Saturated Fat: 0 grams, Carbohydrate: 9 grams, Sugars: 8 grams, Protein: 0 grams, Sodium: 7 milligrams, Cholesterol: 0 milligrams, Fiber: 1 gram, Vitamin D: 0 IU, Calcium: 3 milligrams, Iron: 0 milligrams

Mango-Banana Almond Milk Smoothie

This creamy, dairy-free smoothie is full of fresh, fruity flavor. The potassium, vitamin B6, and other nutrients in the banana and mango make this a healthier and tastier treat than bottled or smoothie-shop drinks.

  8 ounces vanilla almond milk, unsweetened

  1 small **banana**, sliced

  1 cup frozen or fresh mango

Place ingredients in blender and blend until smooth.

▶ **YIELD:** 12 ounces

Nutrition Information per 4 Ounces
Calories: 76, Total Fat: 1 gram, Saturated Fat: 0 grams, Carbohydrate: 17 grams, Sugars: 12 grams, Protein: 1 gram, Sodium: 58 milligrams, Cholesterol: 0 milligrams, Fiber: 2 grams, Vitamin D: 0 IU, Calcium: 150 milligrams, Iron: 0.4 milligrams

Grape Salsa

~~~~~~~~~~

This fresh and fun fruit salsa is perfect for little fingers to eat out of a bowl, on toast, or with cinnamon pita chips. It is packed with manganese for healthy bones and vitamin C for antioxidant power, plus sweet and fruity flavors that kids love. Whole grapes are a no-no for little ones, so halve or quarter them to avoid the choking hazard.

1 cup red seedless **grapes**, quartered

½ cup chopped fresh **pineapple**

½ cup chopped fresh **melon**

1 cup fresh **strawberries**, chopped

½ small **banana**, sliced and quartered

Juice from ½ a **lime**

Combine ingredients in a large bowl and toss to combine. Serve immediately or store in the fridge for up to 2 days.

▶ **YIELD:** 2¾ cups

Nutrition Information per ¼ Cup
Calories: 24, Total Fat: 0 grams, Saturated Fat: 0 grams, Carbohydrate: 6 grams, Sugars: 5 grams, Protein: 0 grams, Sodium: 1 milligram, Cholesterol: 0 milligrams, Fiber: 1 gram, Vitamin D: 0 IU, Calcium: 5 milligrams, Iron: 0.2 milligrams

Cucumbers with Homemade Ranch Dressing

Little appetites are easily pleased with fun finger foods and tasty combos. Skip the bottled salad dressing and make this homemade version to pair with crisp and refreshing cucumbers. Thanks to their high water content, cukes will help keep kids hydrated. If mixing up veggies and dressing is unappealing for your kids, serve the dressing on the side for dunking. This is a good time for good old real mayo, combined with Greek yogurt to cut the fat and boost the protein. This dressing is best when made the night before, as the flavors are enhanced when they sit in the fridge overnight.

¼ cup low-fat buttermilk

2 tablespoons mayonnaise

2 tablespoons nonfat Greek **yogurt**

1 tablespoon chopped fresh **chives**

1 tablespoon chopped fresh **parsley**

1 tablespoon fresh **lemon** juice

½ teaspoon garlic powder

½ teaspoon onion powder

½ teaspoon kosher salt

¼ teaspoon black pepper

1 English **cucumber**, thinly sliced

For the dressing combine buttermilk, mayo, yogurt, herbs, lemon juice, and spices; whisk vigorously. Chill for at least 1 hour before serving. Store in the refrigerator for up to 1 week. Toss cucumbers with dressing or serve on the side for dipping.

▶ **YIELD:** 3 cups cucumber, 2/3 cup dressing

**Nutrition Information per 5 Cucumber Slices and
1 Tablespoon Dressing**
Calories: 30, Total Fat: 2 grams, Saturated Fat: 0 grams, Carbohydrate:
2 grams, Sugars: 0 grams, Protein: 1 gram, Sodium: 147 milligrams,
Cholesterol: 1 milligram, Fiber: 0 grams, Vitamin D: 0 IU, Calcium:
12 milligrams, Iron: 0 milligrams

Roasted Root Vegetables

~~~~~~~~~~~

These veggies are bursting with antioxidants, fiber, and essential nutrients that are vital for growth and development. This simple dish is full of flavor and the perfect accompaniment to any meal. Puree using a food processor or food mill for babies.

1 medium **carrot**, peeled, trimmed, sliced (about ½ cup)

1 medium **potato**, scrubbed, cubed (about 1½ cups)

1 medium **beet**, peeled, cubed (about 1 cup)

1 tablespoon olive oil

¾ teaspoon salt

Preheat oven to 400°F. In a mixing bowl combine carrots, potatoes, and beets. Drizzle with olive oil and salt and mix to combine. Pour onto a greased baking sheet in a single layer. Bake for 20 to 25 minutes, until tender.

▶ **YIELD:** 2 cups

Nutrition Information per ½ Cup
Calories: 94, Total Fat: 4 grams, Saturated Fat: 0 grams, Carbohydrate: 15 grams, Sugars: 3 grams, Protein: 2 grams, Sodium: 251 milligrams, Cholesterol: 0 milligrams, Fiber: 3 grams, Vitamin D: 0 IU, Calcium: 18 milligrams, Iron: 0.8 milligrams

Zucchini Flatbread

~~~~~~~~~

This fun variation on an individual "pizza" is a great way to help encourage your little one to eat their veggies. Calcium-rich mozzarella pairs well with low-calorie summer squash. Once cooked and cooled, cut into slices for little ones to grab and gobble up.

½ cup thinly sliced **zucchini**

½ teaspoon kosher salt

1 tablespoon olive oil

¼ cup marinara sauce (such as Carrot Marinara Sauce, page 68)

1 (6-inch) **whole wheat flatbread** or **pita bread**

¼ cup shredded **mozzarella cheese**

Preheat oven to 375°F. In a mixing bowl combine zucchini, salt, and olive oil; toss well. Spread marinara sauce over flatbread and top with an even layer of zucchini.

Sprinkle with cheese and bake for 12 to 15 minutes, until golden brown and cheese has melted.

▶ **YIELD:** 4 slices

Nutrition Information per Slice
Calories: 104, Total Fat: 6 grams, Saturated Fat: 1 gram, Carbohydrate: 11 grams, Sugars: 2 grams, Protein: 4 grams, Sodium: 493 milligrams, Cholesterol: 4 milligrams, Fiber: 1 gram, Vitamin D: 0 IU, Calcium: 60 milligrams, Iron: 0.8 milligrams

93

Veggie Kebabs

~~~~~~~~~~

This bright, attractive kebab will catch the eye and taste buds of your toddler. Arrange a rainbow of vegetables and send to the grill for a quick sizzle. Just be sure to remove from the skewer before serving.

1 small **yellow bell pepper**, seeded, cored, cut into chunks

1 small **red bell pepper**, seeded, cored, cut into chunks

1 small **green bell pepper**, seeded, cored, cut into chunks

1 small **zucchini**, sliced into ¼-inch rounds

1 large **corn on the cob** (about 8 inches), sliced into 6 pieces

1 tablespoon olive oil

Juice of 1 **lemon**

½ teaspoon kosher salt

Black pepper

Carefully slide vegetables onto skewers, alternating the peppers, zucchini, and corn. In a small bowl, whisk together the olive oil, lemon juice, salt, and pepper. Brush onto skewers. Grill for 10 to 15 minutes, until vegetables are warm and slightly tender.

▶ **YIELD:** 4 kebabs

94

Nutrition Information per ½ Kebab
Calories: 43, Total Fat: 2 grams, Saturated Fat: 0.5 grams, Carbohydrate: 6 grams, Sugars: 2 grams, Protein: 1 gram, Sodium: 150 milligrams, Cholesterol: 0 milligrams, Fiber: 1 gram, Vitamin D: 0 IU, Calcium: 6 milligrams, Iron: 0.2 milligrams

Peachy Parfaits

~~~~~~~~

This playful yet healthy dessert is layered with sweet peaches that contain fiber, vitamin C, and antioxidants, along with calcium from creamy vanilla pudding.

    1 cup low-fat vanilla pudding
    1 large ripe **peach**, peeled, pitted, finely chopped
    ½ cup crushed vanilla wafers (about 10 wafer cookies)
    Whipped cream for topping

In two small parfait glasses or bowls, layer pudding, followed by peaches and cookies; repeat. Cover with plastic wrap and let chill in fridge for 1 to 2 hours. Serve topped with whipped cream.

▶ **YIELD:** 4 servings

Nutrition Information per Serving (About ½ Cup)
Calories: 125, Total Fat: 3 grams, Saturated Fat: 0.5 grams, Carbohydrate: 22 grams, Sugars: 15 grams, Protein: 2 grams, Sodium: 126 milligrams, Cholesterol: 1 milligram, Fiber: 1 gram, Vitamin D: 5 IU, Calcium: 100 milligrams, Iron: 0.5 milligrams

Clementine Dippers

My girls love sweet and tangy clementines—they take such pride in peeling their own, and I know it helps them get their daily dose of vitamins A and C. I'm a huge fan of the combo of citrus and chocolate, but I assumed it would not appeal to tiny palates. I was sorely mistaken! Get the kids in the kitchen to help with the prep of this two-ingredient treat. I also like to add a sprinkle of sea salt on pieces for the grown-ups.

4 ounces dark **chocolate**, finely chopped

6 **clementines**, peeled and separated

Line a baking sheet with parchment paper. Place chocolate in small bowl and melt over a double boiler or in the microwave.* Dip each piece of clementine in chocolate (about halfway) and transfer to baking sheet. Place in the refrigerator for 10 to 12 minutes, until chocolate has hardened. Serve chilled or at room temperature.

* If using the microwave, cook on high in 20- to 30-second increments, stirring well each time.

▶ **YIELD:** about 36 pieces

Nutrition Information per Piece
Calories: 22, Total Fat: 1 gram, Saturated Fat: 1 gram, Carbohydrate: 3 grams, Sugars: 3 grams, Protein: 0 grams, Sodium: 0 milligrams, Cholesterol: 0 milligrams, Fiber: 0 grams, Vitamin D: 0 IU, Calcium: 4 milligrams, Iron: 0.1 milligrams

4

Grain Recipes

· 6 TO 12 MONTHS ·

Baby's First Oatmeal

Simple is best for one of baby's first foods. Babies who are new to solid foods need a more watery consistency; thin out the mixture accordingly and gradually advance to a thicker texture as tolerated.

½ cup rolled **oats**

1 cup water

Additional liquid (water, breast milk, or prepared formula) for thinning out mixture

97

Combine oats and water in a small saucepan. Bring mixture to a boil and reduce to a simmer. Cook for 5 to

6 minutes, until oats are thickened and all the water is absorbed. Remove from heat and allow to cool for at least 10 minutes. Transfer to a food processor and pulse until smooth. When ready to serve, thin out with additional liquid as needed.

▶ **YIELD:** 1 cup

Nutrition Information per ¼ Cup
Calories: 38, Total Fat: 1 gram, Saturated Fat: 0 grams, Carbohydrate: 7 grams, Sugars: 0 grams, Protein: 1 gram, Sodium: 0 milligrams, Cholesterol: 0 milligrams, Fiber: 1 gram, Vitamin D: 0 IU, Calcium: 0 milligrams, Iron: 0.5 milligrams

Brown Rice with Roasted Carrots

~~~~~~~~~

This simple dish is a great way to introduce food combinations. Sweet and tender roasted carrots help balance out the nutty flavor of whole grain brown rice.

    3 large **carrots**, peeled and cut into 1-inch chunks
    1 teaspoon canola oil
    1 cup cooked long-grain **brown rice**
    Water or **stock** (chicken or vegetable)

Preheat oven to 400°F. Place carrots on sheet pan and drizzle with canola oil. Roast for 15 to 20 minutes, until tender. Place carrots and brown rice in a food processor and pulse until mixture is desired consistency. If it appears too dry, add some water or broth and pulse again.

▶ **YIELD:** 1½ cups

Nutrition Information per ¼ Cup
Calories: 55 , Total Fat: 1 gram, Saturated Fat: 0 grams, Carbohydrate: 10 grams, Sugars: 2 grams, Protein: 1 gram, Sodium: 23 milligrams, Cholesterol: 0 milligrams, Fiber: 1 gram, Vitamin D: 0 IU, Calcium: 13 milligrams, Iron: 0.2 milligrams

Whole Grain Pancakes

~~~~~~~~~~

I look forward to lazy weekend breakfasts where we all huddle around the stove to make pancakes. I keep a large batch of the dry ingredients in the pantry at all times to help cut down on prep time. Since most days are not so relaxed, I make lots of extra pancakes and freeze them. You can pop 'em in the microwave straight from the freezer on busy weekday mornings. Babies and toddlers alike love this simple recipe.

1 cup whole **milk**

1 tablespoon white vinegar

1 cup Pancake Mix (see recipe below)

1 large **egg**, lightly beaten

1 teaspoon vanilla extract

2 tablespoons unsalted butter, melted and cooled slightly

Additional butter for greasing pan or griddle

Toppings: butter, fresh **fruit**, jam, **maple syrup**

Combine milk and vinegar in a small bowl or measuring cup, stir and set aside for 5 minutes. In a large bowl, combine pancake mix, milk and vinegar mixture, egg, vanilla, and melted butter; whisk well.

Heat and grease a pan or griddle over medium heat. Pour about 3 tablespoons of batter and cook 2 to 3 minutes per side, until golden brown. Serve with desired toppings.

Pancake Mix (Makes About 3 Cups)

~~~~~~~~~~~~~~~~~~~~~~~~~~~~~~~~~~~

1½ cups **whole wheat pastry flour**

1½ cups all-purpose flour

1 teaspoon baking powder

½ teaspoon baking soda

1½ teaspoons kosher salt

1 tablespoon sugar

▶ **YIELD:** 12 pancakes

Nutrition Information per Pancake
Calories: 70, Total Fat: 3 grams, Saturated Fat: 2 grams, Carbohydrate: 9 grams, Sugars: 2 grams, Protein: 2 grams, Sodium: 130 milligrams, Cholesterol: 7 milligrams, Fiber: 1 gram, Vitamin D: 1 IU, Calcium: 40 milligrams, Iron: 0.4 milligrams

Mac and Cheese with Vegetables and Chicken

~~~~~~~~~~

This is an awesome mixed meal for little ones who are ten to twelve months old. Serve with fruit for a complete and well-balanced meal. I still make this (unpureed) for the entire family to enjoy.

2 cups small-shaped **pasta** (such as stelline or orzo)

½ cup **broccoli** florets

½ cup chopped **carrots**

3 ounces cooked **chicken** breast

¼ cup low-fat **milk**

2 ounces **American cheese**, shredded or chopped (Applegate brand recommended)

Cook pasta according to package directions and set aside. Place broccoli and carrots in a small saucepan and boil until very tender (about 15 minutes). Drain, reserving 1 cup of the cooking liquid. Transfer cooked vegetables and chicken to a food processor and pulse until well chopped; add a bit of reserved veggie cooking liquid if mixture appears too dry. Set aside.

Heat milk in a small saucepan until steamy. Add pasta and cheese; stir with a wooden spoon until well combined. Mix in chicken mixture and add more cooking liquid, if desired.

▶ **YIELD:** about 3 cups

Nutrition Information per ½ Cup
Calories: 147, Total Fat: 4 grams, Saturated Fat: 2 grams, Carbohydrate: 18 grams, Sugars: 1 gram, Protein: 11 grams, Sodium: 157 milligrams, Cholesterol: 21 milligrams, Fiber: 2 grams, Vitamin D: 5 IU, Calcium: 78 milligrams, Iron: 0.6 milligrams

Dressed-Up Frozen Waffles with Pears and Honey

~~~~~~~~~

You don't always have to make breakfast from scratch. On super busy mornings pop a whole grain waffle in the toaster. Make it special and boost the fiber with a 1-minute sauce.

1 frozen **whole grain waffle**, toasted

1 **pear**, peeled and chopped

1 teaspoon **honey**

While waffle is toasting, prepare the sauce. Place chopped pear and honey in a small bowl. Microwave on high for 1 minute, until pear is tender. Stir and allow to cool for 5 minutes. Pour sauce over toasted waffle or on the side for dipping.

▶ **YIELD:** 1 waffle

Nutrition Information per ½ Waffle (with Topping)
Calories: 98, Total Fat: 1 gram, Saturated Fat: 0 grams, Carbohydrate: 24 grams, Sugars: 13 grams, Protein: 1 gram, Sodium: 99 milligrams, Cholesterol: 0 milligrams, Fiber: 3 grams, Vitamin D: 0 IU, Calcium: 19 milligrams, Iron: 1 milligram

Blueberry–Greek Yogurt Mini Muffins

Lots of superfoods make tasty muffins, but blueberries are a top pick. We grab muffins for breakfast on the go or as a light snack. I often bring a big batch into preschool for a class treat. They freeze well, so make ahead, store in the freezer, and defrost as needed.

1 cup unbleached organic all-purpose flour

1 cup **whole wheat pastry flour**

2 teaspoons baking soda

½ teaspoon kosher salt

½ cup **maple syrup**

1 **egg**, beaten

¼ cup canola oil

½ cup plain nonfat Greek **yogurt**

1 teaspoon pure vanilla extract

1 cup low-fat **milk**

2 cups **blueberries**

2 teaspoons **lemon** zest

Preheat oven to 350°F. Spray a mini muffin pan with nonstick cooking spray. In a large bowl, whisk flours, baking soda, and salt.

In a separate bowl whisk together maple syrup, egg, canola oil, Greek yogurt, vanilla, and milk. Add yogurt mixture to dry ingredients, mix until just combined. Gently fold in blueberries and lemon zest. Using a tablespoon, scoop batter into muffin pan. Bake for 8 minutes or until a toothpick comes out clean from the center.

104

▶ **YIELD:** 36 mini muffins

Nutrition Information per Muffin
Calories: 60, Total Fat: 2 grams, Saturated Fat: 0 grams, Carbohydrate: 10 grams, Sugars: 4 grams, Protein: 1 gram, Sodium: 95 milligrams, Cholesterol: 5 milligrams, Fiber: 1 gram, Vitamin D: 5 IU, Calcium: 15 milligrams, Iron: 0.3 milligrams

Three-Cheese Pizza

～～～～～

Pizza is a blank canvas for superfoods, and every Friday is pizza night in our house. It makes for an easy dinner that everyone looks forward to at the end of a busy week. Make batches of dough ahead and store in the freezer. Make sure to get the kids in the kitchen to help choose the toppings and sprinkle the cheese.

1 batch Homemade Pizza Dough (see recipe below) or store-bought dough at room temperature

2 tablespoons olive oil

½ cup marinara sauce (such as Carrot Marinara Sauce, page 68)

8 slices **provolone cheese**

8 ounces shredded part-skim **mozzarella cheese**

¼ cup grated **Parmesan cheese**

Topping suggestions: olives, **bell peppers**, uncured turkey pepperoni (such as Applegate), sliced tomato

Place a large baking sheet or pizza pan in the oven to warm. Turn dough out onto a lightly floured surface and roll flat using a rolling pin. Carefully remove pan from oven and drizzle with olive oil. Transfer dough to pan and gently press to the edges. Top with marinara, cheese, and additional toppings, if desired. Bake for 14 to 15 minutes, turning pan once halfway through cooking. Allow to cool slightly before slicing.

Homemade Pizza Dough

(Makes 1¾-Pound-Piece of Dough)

~~~~~~~~~~~~~~~~~~~~~~~~~~~~~~~~

1 package dry active yeast

1 teaspoon sugar

1 cup warm water

2 cups all-purpose flour

1 cup bread flour or **whole wheat pastry flour**

2 teaspoons kosher salt

Extra virgin olive oil

Combine yeast, sugar, and water in a large measuring cup and whisk to combine. Allow to rest for 10 minutes, until foamy. Place flours and salt in the bowl of an electric mixer fitted with a dough hook. Add the yeast mixture and 1 tablespoon of olive oil. Run machine on low until ingredients are just combined. Increase speed to medium for 6 to 8 minutes, until dough has come together in a large ball. Transfer dough to an oiled bowl and cover with a clean kitchen towel. Let rise for at least 1 hour.

▶ **YIELD:** 12 large or 24 small slices

Nutrition Information per 1 Small Slice
Calories: 119, Total Fat: 5 grams, Saturated Fat: 3 grams, Carbohydrate: 12 grams, Sugars: 1 gram, Protein: 7 grams, Sodium: 247 milligrams, Cholesterol: 15 milligrams, Fiber: 0 grams, Vitamin D: 1.3 IU, Calcium: 152 milligrams, Iron: 0.7 milligrams

Cheesy Rice with Peas

~~~~~~

Some children may be turned off by the flaky texture of cooked rice. Adding something soft and sticky (in a good way) like cheese helps make it easier to eat. This recipe is also my answer to those high-sodium boxed rice mixes with the seasoning packets.

1 cup **brown rice**

2 cups water

1 tablespoon canola oil

2 packets Latin spice mix seasoning (such as no-salt-added Goya Sazón Natural & Complete)

1 tablespoon freshly squeezed **lemon** juice

1 cup frozen green **peas**

¾ cup low-fat shredded **cheddar cheese**

In a 3-quart saucepan or Dutch oven, combine rice and water. Bring to a boil, cover, and reduce heat and simmer until rice is tender (30–35 minutes). In a small bowl, combine canola oil, spice mix, and lemon juice; stir to combine and set aside. When the rice is cooked, add the spice mixture, peas, and cheese; mix well and serve.

▶ **YIELD:** about 4 cups

Nutrition Information per ½ Cup
Calories: 136, Total Fat: 3 grams, Saturated Fat: 1 gram, Carbohydrate: 20 grams, Sugars: 1 gram, Protein: 6 grams, Sodium: 181 milligrams, Cholesterol: 3 milligrams, Fiber: 2 grams, Vitamin D: 1 IU, Calcium: 56 milligrams, Iron: 0.5 milligrams

Whole Grain Chocolate Cupcakes with Cream Cheese and Mascarpone Frosting

I am always on a mission to make from-scratch baked goods. These cupcakes have become my go-to recipe for birthday parties, holidays, and weekends when I feel like making special treats. Whole wheat pastry flour adds some whole grain goodness, and the preservative, and trans-fat-free icing is a healthier blank canvas for any kind of decorations.

1 cup **whole wheat pastry flour**

1 cup all-purpose flour

1 cup unsweetened **cocoa** powder

1½ teaspoons baking soda

½ teaspoon salt

1 stick unsalted butter

1⅓ cups sugar

⅓ cup light brown sugar

2 large **eggs**

2 teaspoons vanilla extract

1 cup whole **milk**

¼ cup water

Cream Cheese and Mascarpone Frosting (recipe below)

Preheat oven to 350°F. Line a 12-cup muffin pan with paper liners. Sift together flours, cocoa powder, baking soda, and salt; set aside. In the bowl of an electric stand mixer fitted with a paddle attachment, cream together butter and both sugars until fluffy (2–3 minutes). With the mixer on low, add the eggs, one at a time, followed by the vanilla. Alternately add the dry ingredients and the milk and water until all ingredients are well mixed. Using an ice-cream scoop or ¼ cup measure, place batter into pans and bake for 17 to 20 minutes or until a toothpick inserted in the center comes out clean. Let cool completely and top with frosting. Decorate as desired.

Cream Cheese and Mascarpone Frosting

8 ounces cream cheese, softened

8 ounces ⅓ reduced fat cream cheese, softened (aka Neufchâtel)

4 tablespoons unsalted butter, softened

¼ cup **mascarpone cheese**

1 teaspoon vanilla extract

3 cups confectioners' sugar

In a medium bowl, combine cream cheeses, butter, mascarpone, and vanilla. Using an electric mixer, blend ingredients together while slowly adding confectioners' sugar in batches. Continue to beat until smooth and creamy. Frosting can be made ahead and stored in the refrigerator for up to 3 days. Allow it to sit out for 10 to 15 minutes before frosting cupcakes.

▶ **YIELD:** 24 cupcakes

Nutrition Information per 1 Cupcake with Frosting
Calories: 227, Total Fat: 14 grams, Saturated Fat: 8 grams, Carbohydrate: 24 grams, Sugars: 15 grams, Protein: 4 grams, Sodium: 185 milligrams, Cholesterol: 51 milligrams, Fiber: 2 grams, Vitamin D: 10 IU, Calcium: 37 milligrams, Iron: 1.4 milligrams

Nut-Free Granola

~~~~~~~~

This no-fail granola recipe is better than anything out of a box. Once potential allergies have been ruled out, add pumpkin seeds or sesame seeds for some extra crunch. Dried cranberries are a tasty pairing with the coconut, but dried apricots, raisins, and cherries work well too. Some children have trouble with chewy dried fruits, so consider chopping finely before adding to the mix.

2½ cups rolled **oats**

½ cup sweetened shredded **coconut**

¼ teaspoon kosher salt

⅓ cup **maple syrup** or agave nectar

1 tablespoon canola oil

1 cup dried **cranberries**

Preheat oven to 300°F. Spray a large baking sheet with nonstick cooking spray. Combine oats, coconut, salt, maple syrup, and canola oil in a large bowl. Toss well and transfer to prepared baking sheet. Bake, stirring occasionally, until golden brown (15–20 minutes). Remove from oven. Once cool, mix in dried cranberries. Store in an airtight container for up to 1 week.

▶ **YIELD:** 3½ cups

111

Nutrition Information per ¼ Cup
Calories: 128, Total Fat: 4 grams, Saturated Fat: 2 grams, Carbohydrate: 22 grams, Sugars: 12 grams, Protein: 2 grams, Sodium: 33 milligrams, Cholesterol: 0 milligrams, Fiber: 2 grams, Vitamin D: 0 IU, Calcium: 8 milligrams, Iron: 0.7 milligrams

Breakfast Quinoa with Cherries

This oatmeal alternative will get kids to fall in love with quinoa. It's higher in protein and fiber than oatmeal and contains all of the building blocks that tiny muscles need. Use fresh cherries when they're in season and opt for dried or frozen when they're not.

1 cup low-fat **milk** or almond milk
½ cup **quinoa**
Pinch of kosher salt
1 teaspoon light brown sugar or turbinado sugar
½ cup fresh or dried cherries

Bring milk to a simmer in a small saucepan. Add quinoa, salt, and sugar. Reduce heat and cook until quinoa is tender and liquid is absorbed (12–15 minutes). Stir in cherries and allow to sit for at least 5 minutes before serving.

▶ **YIELD:** about 1⅓ cups

Nutrition Information per ⅓ Cup
Calories: 128, Total Fat: 2 grams, Saturated Fat: 1 gram, Carbohydrate: 23 grams, Sugars: 8 grams, Protein: 5 grams, Sodium: 67 milligrams, Cholesterol: 4 milligrams, Fiber: 2 grams, Vitamin D: 25 IU, Calcium: 85 milligrams, Iron: 1 milligram

Charlie's Double Pumpkin Muffins

~~~~~~~~

Charlotte is obsessed with pumpkin muffins, and there are no complaints from me. I created this recipe especially with her in mind, and I find myself making and freezing batches of these at least once a month. Pumpkin seeds make for the "double" pumpkin designation, but sometimes we just make them plain. They are also dynamite when you add a couple handfuls of mini chocolate chips to the batter.

1 cup all-purpose flour

1 cup **whole wheat pastry flour**

1½ teaspoons baking powder

½ teaspoon baking soda

½ teaspoon ground cinnamon

1 teaspoon kosher salt

1 cup light brown sugar

1 large **egg**, beaten

½ cup canola oil

1 (3-ounce) pouch carrot-applesauce (Trader Joe's Crushers recommended)

¼ cup whole **milk**

1 teaspoon vanilla extract

1 cup canned **pumpkin** puree

Pumpkin seeds and sparkling sugar

Preheat oven to 375°F. Spray mini muffin pan with non-stick cooking spray and set aside. In a large bowl, combine flours, baking powder, baking soda, cinnamon, and salt; whisk well to combine. In a separate bowl whisk together brown sugar, egg, canola oil, carrot-applesauce, milk, vanilla, and pumpkin puree. Add pumpkin mixture to dry ingredients and mix until just combined. Fill each muffin cup with 1 tablespoon of batter and sprinkle with pumpkin seeds and sparkling sugar. Bake for 12 to 14 minutes or until a toothpick comes out clean from the center. Allow to cool for at least 20 minutes before serving.

▶ **YIELD:** 36 mini muffins

Nutrition Information per Muffin
Calories: 77, Total Fat: 3 grams, Saturated Fat: 0 grams, Carbohydrate: 11 grams, Sugars: 6 grams, Protein: 1 gram, Sodium: 73 milligrams, Cholesterol: 5 milligrams, Fiber: 1 gram, Vitamin D: 1 IU, Calcium: 7 milligrams, Iron: 0.3 milligrams

Whole Grain Pita Chips with Edamame Hummus

~~~~~~~~

This protein-packed dip is super fun for dunking veg-gies and homemade pita chips—they're healthier than anything out of a bag! For thinner chips, use whole wheat flour tortillas.

3 (6-inch) **whole wheat pitas**

4 tablespoons olive oil, divided

¾ teaspoon kosher salt

⅛ teaspoon black pepper, plus more to taste

2 cups shelled frozen **edamame**, thawed

2 tablespoons whipped cream cheese

1 tablespoon **honey**

Juice and zest of 1 **lemon**

Preheat oven to 350°F. Using a sharp knife or pizza cutter, slice each pita into eight triangles. Place 1 tablespoon olive oil in a small bowl, season with ¼ teaspoon salt and pepper (to taste). Place pita wedges on a large sheet pan and brush with seasoned oil. Bake for 5 to 7 minutes or until they just begin to turn golden brown. While chips are baking, make the dip. Place edamame, remaining oil, cream cheese, honey, lemon juice and zest, ½ teaspoon salt, and ⅛ teaspoon pepper in a food processor and run until smooth and creamy. Serve dip with chips on the side.

▶ **YIELD:** 24 chips and 1¾ cups dip

Nutrition Information per Serving (3 Chips and 1 Tablespoon Dip)
Calories: 95, Total Fat: 3 grams, Saturated Fat: 0 grams, Carbohydrate: 15 grams, Sugars: 1 gram, Protein: 4 grams, Sodium: 187 milligrams, Cholesterol: 1 milligram, Fiber: 2 grams, Vitamin D: 0 IU, Calcium: 11 milligrams, Iron: 1 milligram

French Toast Sticks with Blackberry Sauce

Growing up, I loved making French toast with my parents on the weekends. It means so much to me to make this version with my own kids. Cutting it into sticks makes it easier for tiny fingers to enjoy. The purple dipping sauce is pretty popular too!

2 cups fresh or frozen **blackberries**

¼ cup water

¼ cup 100 percent **maple syrup**

1 tablespoon fresh **lemon** juice

1 large **egg**

½ cup low-fat (1 percent) **milk**

½ teaspoon pure vanilla extract

1 teaspoon ground cinnamon, plus more to taste

1 tablespoon unsalted butter or Smart Balance Buttery Spread, divided

3 slices **whole grain bread**

For the blackberry sauce: Combine berries, water, maple syrup, and lemon juice in a small saucepan. Heat over medium heat until bubbly and berries begin to break down (about 10 minutes). Transfer mixture to a food processor fitted with a steel blade. Pulse until smooth, strain through a fine mesh strainer to remove seeds. Set aside to cool.

For the French toast: In a large bowl, whisk together egg, milk, vanilla, and cinnamon; set aside. Heat a large nonstick skillet over medium heat; spray with nonstick spray. Melt half the butter in the skillet. Dip two slices of bread into milk mixture, making sure both sides are well coated. Place bread in skillet and cook for 2 to 3 minutes per side or until golden brown (sprinkle with additional cinnamon, if desired). Repeat with remaining slice of bread. Cool slightly and cut each slice into four sticks. Serve with blackberry sauce.

▶ **YIELD:** 12 sticks and ⅔ cup sauce

**Nutrition Information per Serving
(3 Sticks and 2 Tablespoons Sauce)**
Calories: 230, Total Fat: 5 grams, Saturated Fat: 1 gram, Carbohydrate: 41 grams, Sugars: 24 grams, Protein: 6 grams, Sodium: 202 milligrams, Cholesterol: 48 milligrams, Fiber: 5 grams, Vitamin D: 38 IU, Calcium: 204 milligrams, Iron: 2 milligrams

Arugula Pesto Pasta

Affectionately called "green macaroni," this quick and easy creation makes its way onto our table for weeknight dinners and holiday celebrations alike. You can turn just about any kind of leafy green vegetable or herb into pesto; nutrient-filled arugula is one of the most popular in our house. Make large batches to store in the fridge and freezer so it's ready to go when you are.

1 pound rotini **pasta**

¼ cup heavy cream

¼ cup Arugula Pesto (recipe below) or use prepared pesto from the grocery store

Cook pasta according to package directions. Drain and set aside. In the same pot add cream and bring to a simmer. Stir in pesto (if frozen, can be added straight from the freezer). Stir and cook for 2 to 3 minutes, until slightly thickened. Add pasta and toss to coat.

Arugula Pesto (Makes 1½ cups)

4 cups fresh arugula

1 clove garlic, chopped

Juice and zest of 1 **lemon**

¼ cup grated **Parmesan cheese** (optional)

1 teaspoon kosher salt

Black pepper

¾ cup extra virgin olive oil

Combine arugula, garlic, lemon juice and zest, Parmesan (if using), salt, and pepper (to taste) in a food processor fitted with a steel blade. Pulse until smooth. With the machine on, slowly pour in olive oil. Blend until smooth. Serve immediately, refrigerate for up to 1 week, or freeze for up to 3 months.

▶ **YIELD:** 8 cups

Nutrition Information per ½ Cup
Calories: 134, Total Fat: 4 grams, Saturated Fat: 1 gram, Carbohydrate: 21 grams, Sugars: 1 gram, Protein: 4 grams, Sodium: 19 milligrams, Cholesterol: 5 milligrams, Fiber: 1 gram, Vitamin D: 1 IU, Calcium: 13 milligrams, Iron: 1 milligram

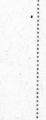

Banana Chocolate Chip Bread

~~~~~~~~~~

There's no better way to use up overripe bananas! This recipe is incredibly flexible—use applesauce instead of apple butter or almond milk instead of soy (cow's milk works too), and it still comes out perfect every time. This banana bread is also allergy-friendly because it's free of eggs and nuts. You can eliminate any traces of dairy by using vegan chocolate chips, or swap out gluten-free baking mix for the flour. I prefer to make this in a large Bundt pan or mini loaves.* If you use a standard loaf pan, you'll have some extra batter left over for some muffins.

3/4 cup **maple syrup**

1/4 cup **honey**

2 ripe **bananas**, mashed

1 teaspoon cinnamon

1/4 teaspoon freshly grated nutmeg

1/4 cup canola oil

1/4 cup apple butter

1 teaspoon pure vanilla extract

1 cup unsweetened soy milk

1 cup all-purpose flour

1 cup **whole wheat pastry flour**

2 teaspoons baking soda

1/2 teaspoon kosher salt

1 cup semisweet **chocolate** chips

Preheat oven to 350°F. Spray a loaf pan with nonstick cooking spray and set aside. In a large saucepan, combine maple syrup, honey, bananas, cinnamon, nutmeg, canola oil, apple butter, vanilla, and soy milk. Heat over low heat for 2 to 3 minutes; whisk to combine and set aside to cool for 15 minutes. In a large bowl, combine flours, baking soda, and salt; set aside. Add banana mixture to dry ingredients; mix until just combined. Make sure batter has cooled, then stir in the chocolate chips. Pour batter into prepared loaf pan and bake for 45 to 50 minutes or until a toothpick comes out clean from the center. Allow to cool for at least 30 minutes before serving.

* If using a Bundt pan, increase cooking time to 55 to 60 minutes.

▶ **YIELD:** 12 large or 24 small slices

Nutrition Information per 1 Small Slice
Calories: 156, Total Fat: 5 grams, Saturated Fat: 2 grams, Carbohydrate: 27 grams, Sugars: 17 grams, Protein: 2 grams, Sodium: 133 milligrams, Cholesterol: 0 milligrams, Fiber: 1 gram, Vitamin D: 5 IU, Calcium: 25 milligrams, Iron: 0.4 milligrams

Cinnamon Roll Oatmeal

I've made oatmeal this way so many times I had to write up the recipe. It has all the sweet goodness of sticky buns, but it is a much healthier way to start your day. For easy morning time prep, make plain oatmeal ahead and store in the fridge. Microwave to reheat and then pile on the toppings.

- 1 teaspoon ground cinnamon
- 4 teaspoons brown sugar
- 1½ cups rolled **oats**
- ¼ cup **raisins**
- ¼ cup chopped walnuts (optional)
- Low-fat **milk** or soy milk (optional)

In a small bowl, combine cinnamon and sugar—set aside. Prepare oats with water according to package directions. Top with cinnamon, sugar, and raisins, and walnuts, if using; stir. Finish with a splash of milk or soy milk, if desired.

▶ **YIELD:** 3 cups

Nutrition Information per ½ Cup
Calories: 143, Total Fat: 5 grams, Saturated Fat: 1 gram, Carbohydrate: 24 grams, Sugars: 13 grams, Protein: 3 grams, Sodium: 64 milligrams, Cholesterol: 0 milligrams, Fiber: 2 grams, Vitamin D: 17 IU, Calcium: 25 milligrams, Iron: 1.7 milligrams

Real Microwave Popcorn

~~~~~~~~

Save time and money and skip all those preservatives. Making real microwave popcorn is so easy that my daughter taught our babysitter how to do it. Season freshly popped popcorn with cinnamon sugar, Parmesan cheese, fresh herbs, or cocoa powder. Popcorn can be a choking hazard, so be sure to give small serving sizes, especially the first few times you serve it to the younger kids.

    ¼ cup **popcorn** kernels

    1 tablespoon buttery spread such as Smart Balance, melted

    Kosher salt to taste

Place kernels in a brown paper lunch bag and fold over the top twice to close. Microwave on high for approximately 2 minutes. Pour into a large bowl and top with melted buttery spread and season with salt.

▶ **YIELD:** 6 cups

Nutrition Information per 1 Cup
Calories: 40, Total Fat: 2 grams, Saturated Fat: 0 grams, Carbohydrate: 6 grams, Sugars: 0 grams, Protein: 1 gram, Sodium: 108 milligrams, Cholesterol: 0 milligrams, Fiber: 1 gram, Vitamin D: 0 IU, Calcium: 0 milligrams, Iron: 0.4 milligrams

123

Slow-Cooker Coconut Rice

I love to use my slow cooker for more than just one-pot meals. Throw the ingredients for this healthy and tasty side dish in the Crock-Pot and head to the park for the afternoon. Serve with grilled chicken or shrimp and steamed veggies.

1 cup dry long-grain **brown rice**

1 can light **coconut** milk (about 2 cups)

1 cup water

1 teaspoon kosher salt

Combine ingredients in a slow cooker and stir. Cover and cook on high for 2 hours.

▶ **YIELD:** 3½ cups

Nutrition Information per ¼ Cup
Calories: 75, Total Fat: 3 grams, Saturated Fat: 2 grams, Carbohydrate: 11 grams, Sugars: 1 gram, Protein: 1 gram, Sodium: 88 milligrams, Cholesterol: 0 milligrams, Fiber: 0 grams, Vitamin D: 0 IU, Calcium: 9 milligrams, Iron: 0.3 milligrams

Peanut Butter Spaghetti

Peanut butter for dinner! This Asian-inspired noodle dish is high in protein and healthy fats. Kids just can't get enough of it. Leftover sauce makes a tasty dip for chicken or veggie sticks.

12 ounces dry **spaghetti**

1 clove garlic

½ cup creamy **peanut butter**

¼ cup reduced-sodium soy sauce

2 tablespoons **honey**

2 tablespoons sherry or rice vinegar

1 tablespoon canola oil

1 teaspoon sesame oil

Shredded **carrots** and thinly sliced **cucumber** for serving

Cook pasta according to package directions; drain, reserving ¼ cup of the cooking liquid. While the pasta is cooking, prepare the sauce. Add garlic to food processor and pulse to finely chop. Add peanut butter, soy sauce, honey, vinegar, canola and sesame oils; pulse until smooth. With the machine running, add reserved cooking liquid through the feed tube. Toss ½ cup of prepared sauce with cooked pasta. Serve with carrots and cucumbers on top or on the side.

▶ **YIELD:** 6 cups

Nutrition Information per ½ Cup
Calories: 197, Total Fat: 8 grams, Saturated Fat: 1 gram, Carbohydrate: 25 grams, Sugars: 4 grams, Protein: 8 grams, Sodium: 230 milligrams, Cholesterol: 0 milligrams, Fiber: 1 gram, Vitamin D: 0 IU, Calcium: 13 milligrams, Iron: 1.4 milligrams

Chocolate-Dipped Pretzels

These crunchy, sweet, and salty treats are my top pick for class parties, bake sales, and holiday treats. Use chips or chopped bars of chocolate (whatever's in the pantry); you can make a huge batch of these in less than 30 minutes.

8 ounces semisweet **chocolate**

8 ounces white **chocolate**

1 bag salted pretzel rods

Assorted sprinkles and colored sugar

Line two baking sheets with parchment paper. Place chocolate in a bowl and melt over a double boiler or in the microwave.* Pour melted chocolate into a tall drinking glass. Tilt the glass downward slightly, being careful not to spill the chocolate. Then dip and roll the pretzel in chocolate to coat; transfer to baking sheet and sprinkle with colored sugar or other desired decorations. Allow to set for at least 30 minutes or until chocolate has hardened. Store in cellophane or resealable plastic bags.

* If using the microwave, cook on high in 20- to 30-second increments, stirring well each time.

▶ **YIELD:** 30 pieces

Nutrition Information per Piece
Calories: 100, Total Fat: 4 grams, Saturated Fat: 2 grams, Carbohydrate: 15 grams, Sugars: 7 grams, Protein: 2 grams, Sodium: 208 milligrams, Cholesterol: 1 milligram, Fiber: 1 gram, Vitamin D: 0 IU, Calcium: 11 milligrams, Iron: 0.5 milligrams

5

Protein Recipes

· 6 TO 12 MONTHS ·

Easy Chicken Soup

Boxed chicken broth can be a huge time saver, but there's nothing as delicious as homemade chicken stock. It is rich in vitamins and minerals, plus it helps keep kids hydrated. Keep quarts at the ready in the freezer to make soups, sauces, and risotto on the fly. I love to make batches of this soup to deliver to family and friends when they're feeling under the weather.

1 quart Homemade Chicken Stock (recipe below)

1 cup mixed frozen vegetables (**peas**, **green beans**, **corn**, and **carrots**)

2/3 cup cooked **brown rice** or **pasta**

Bring stock to a boil in a medium saucepan. Add vegetables and rice or pasta and simmer until all ingredients are heated through. For children ages nine to twelve months, puree to desired texture.

▶ **YIELD:** 1 quart

Homemade Chicken Stock (Makes 3 Quarts)

1 (3- to 4-pound) whole **chicken**

1 white **onion**, quartered

2 large **carrots**, roughly chopped

2 large celery stalks, roughly chopped

2 cloves garlic

2 handfuls **fresh herbs** (such as parsley, basil, dill, thyme, tarragon, and rosemary)

1 tablespoon kosher salt

1 teaspoon black peppercorns

2 bay leaves

1 gallon water

Place chicken in the bottom of a large (5- or 6-quart) stockpot. Toss in onion, carrots, celery, garlic, herbs, salt, peppercorns, and bay leaves. Add enough water to cover (about 1 gallon). Bring to a boil uncovered, reduce to a simmer, and cook for 3 hours. Strain and transfer to plastic or glass containers. Store in the refrigerator for up to 1 week or in the freezer for up to 6 months.

Nutrition Information per 1 Cup
Calories: 33, Total Fat: 2 grams, Saturated Fat: 1 gram, Carbohydrate: 0 grams, Sugars: 0 grams, Protein: 4 grams, Sodium: 381 milligrams, Cholesterol: 12 milligrams, Fiber: 0 grams, Vitamin D: 0 IU, Calcium: 12 milligrams, Iron: 0.2 milligrams

Pork and Potatoes

~~~~~~

A balanced meal with each spoonful, this combination of meat, starch, and veggie is baby's first intro to a "grown-up" dinner. Pork is an excellent source of thiamin, an energy-producing B vitamin, and the creaminess of the mineral-rich potatoes helps make it easier to enjoy.

   1 large bone-in **pork** chop (about 6 ounces)
   1 medium **potato**, peeled and diced
   1 cup frozen **peas**

Place pork chop and potato in a medium saucepan. Cover with water and bring to a low boil. Reduce heat to medium and cook for 40 to 45 minutes, turn off heat, and add peas.* Transfer to a bowl to cool slightly, reserving 1 cup of the cooking liquid. Remove meat from the bone and transfer it along with potatoes and peas to a food processor and pulse until the mixture is well combined but still has some texture. Add a few splashes of cooking liquid to make the mixture smoother, if desired. Store in the refrigerator for up to 3 days or transfer to ice cube trays and freeze for up to 3 months.

   * To ensure that the meat is thoroughly cooked, use a meat thermometer; the proper internal temperature for pork is 145°F to 150°F.

129

▶ **YIELD:** about 2 cups

Nutrition Information per ¼ Cup
Calories: 61, Total Fat: 1 gram, Saturated Fat: 0 grams, Carbohydrate: 7 grams, Sugars: 1 gram, Protein: 6 grams, Sodium: 17 milligrams, Cholesterol: 15 milligrams, Fiber: 1 gram, Vitamin D: 3 IU, Calcium: 7 milligrams, Iron: 0.5 milligrams

Chicken Thighs with Sweet Potato

~~~

Dark-meat poultry gets a bad reputation for being too high in fat, but it is actually rich in healthy unsaturated fats that are vital for baby's growth and development. Dark meat also contains more iron than white meat. The natural sugars in sweet potatoes make this dish extra pleasing for tiny taste buds.

3 large, bone-in **chicken** thighs
1 large **sweet potato**, peeled and diced

Place chicken thighs and sweet potato in a medium saucepan. Cover with water and bring to a low boil. Reduce heat to medium and cook for 30 to 35 minutes.* Transfer to a bowl to cool slightly, reserving 1 cup of the cooking liquid. Remove meat from the bone and transfer it along with sweet potato to a food processor and pulse until the mixture is well combined but still has some texture. Add a few splashes of cooking liquid to make the mixture smoother, if desired. Store in the refrigerator for up to 3 days or transfer to ice cube trays and freeze for up to 3 months.

* To ensure that the meat is thoroughly cooked, use a meat thermometer; the proper internal temperature for chicken is 165°F.

▶ **YIELD:** about 1½ cups

Nutrition Information per ¼ Cup
Calories: 60, Total Fat: 1 gram, Saturated Fat: 0 grams, Carbohydrate: 4 grams, Sugars: 1 gram, Protein: 7 grams, Sodium: 42 milligrams, Cholesterol: 29 milligrams, Fiber: 1 gram, Vitamin D: 2 IU, Calcium: 10 milligrams, Iron: 0.5 milligrams

Deconstructed Broccoli and Tofu Stir-Fry

Two superfoods take center stage in this crowd-pleasing dish. A mound of mixed food like typically seen in stir-fry can be a little overwhelming to young children, so much so that it might deter them from even tasting it. Try separating the components on the plate. Chop into tiny bites for ages twelve to eighteen months. Serve it with brown rice or rice noodles.

½ block extra-firm **tofu** (7 ounces)

2 tablespoons canola oil, divided

2 tablespoons low-sodium soy sauce, divided

1 teaspoon freshly grated ginger

3 cups **broccoli** florets

Preheat oven to 425°F. Slice tofu into pieces approximately ½ inch thick and 2 inches long (domino-size pieces). Place pieces on a flat surface lined with a paper towel and press down gently to remove excess water. Place tofu pieces on a sheet pan, drizzle with 1 tablespoon each canola oil and soy sauce; toss well to coat. Bake for 20 to 25 minutes (turning once), until golden brown. Heat remaining oil in a large skillet or wok, add ginger and allow to cook for about 25 seconds. Add broccoli and remaining soy sauce. Stir-fry until broccoli is just cooked (about 7 minutes).

131

▶ **YIELD:** about 6 cups

Nutrition Information per 1 Cup
Calories: 109, Total Fat: 8 grams, Saturated Fat: 0 grams, Carbohydrate:
5 grams, Sugars: 2 grams, Protein: 7 grams, Sodium: 120 milligrams,
Cholesterol: 0 milligrams, Fiber: 2 grams, Vitamin D: 0 IU, Calcium:
241 milligrams, Iron: 1 milligram

~~~~~~~~~~~~~~

Baked Bison Meatballs

Yup, bison! Low in fat but high in protein, iron, and omega-3 fats. The low fat content means that the meat can dry out easily, but the cooking method and the secret ingredient (balsamic onions) keep these babies moist and flavorful. You can also use this recipe using 90 percent lean ground turkey or lean ground beef. I like to serve them with pasta or solo with some marinara or barbecue sauce for dipping.

2 teaspoons olive oil

¼ cup finely chopped red onion

Kosher salt and black pepper

2 teaspoons balsamic vinegar

1 pound ground **bison**

1 large **egg**, beaten

2 tablespoons **whole wheat panko bread crumbs**

2 tablespoons Italian-seasoned bread crumbs

2 tablespoons chopped fresh **parsley** or 1 tablespoon Arugula Pesto (page 118)

Heat olive oil in a small skillet. Add onion, season to taste with salt and pepper, and cook for 2 minutes. Add balsamic vinegar and cook for an additional 5 minutes. Remove from heat and set aside to cool. Preheat oven to 350°F. Line a baking sheet with parchment paper. In a large bowl, combine ground bison, cooked onions, egg, bread crumbs, and parsley (or pesto, if using). Season with an additional ½ teaspoon each salt and pepper. With clean hands, gently mix well and form into sixteen 1-ounce balls. Transfer to lined baking sheet

133

and bake for 20 to 25 minutes. Use a meat thermometer to ensure the proper internal temperature. The USDA recommendation for ground meat is 160°F to 165°F.

▶ **YIELD:** 16 meatballs

Nutrition Information per Meatball
Calories: 58, Total Fat: 3 grams, Saturated Fat: 1 gram, Carbohydrate: 1 gram, Sugars: 0 grams, Protein: 6 grams, Sodium: 94 milligrams, Cholesterol: 27 milligrams, Fiber: 0 grams, Vitamin D: 3 IU, Calcium: 8 milligrams, Iron: 1 milligram

Teriyaki Pork Tenderloin

Lean pork tenderloin is a wonderful source of protein. The teriyaki marinade helps to tenderize the meat so it is never tough or chewy. Since pork tenderloins are typically sold in two-packs, I'll double this recipe and prepare them both. Leftovers are great for sandwiches, quesadillas, or diced and tossed with rice and stir-fried vegetables.

- ¼ cup reduced-sodium soy sauce
- 1 clove garlic, minced
- 1-inch piece ginger root, peeled and finely chopped
- 2 tablespoons brown sugar
- 1 tablespoon rice vinegar
- 1 pound **pork** tenderloin, trimmed

Place soy sauce, garlic, ginger, brown sugar, and vinegar in a large resealable plastic bag. Add pork, transfer to the refrigerator, and marinate for at least 30 minutes or up to 8 hours. Preheat a grill or grill pan over medium heat. Remove pork from marinade (discard marinade) and cook for 3 to 4 minutes per side or until internal temperature reaches 145°F to 150°F. Let rest for 10 minutes before slicing.

Preparation variation: Instead of grilling, sear on all sides in an oven-safe skillet and transfer to a 425°F oven. Roast until internal temperature reaches 145°F to 150°F.

▶ **YIELD:** 1 pork tenderloin

135

Nutrition Information per 2 Ounces Cooked Pork
Calories: 70, Total Fat: 1 gram, Saturated Fat: 0 grams, Carbohydrate: 2 grams, Sugars: 2 grams, Protein: 12 grams, Sodium: 110 milligrams, Cholesterol: 37 milligrams, Fiber: 0 grams, Vitamin D: 5 IU, Calcium: 3 milligrams, Iron: 0.6 milligrams

Slow-Cooker Lentil Soup

~~~~~~~~~~

This flavorful, protein- and veggie-packed soup is so delicious your kiddies will want seconds. For extra flavor and calcium, top servings with a sprinkle of their favorite cheese.

2¼ cups dry green **lentils**

2 tablespoons olive oil

1 tablespoon butter

1 tablespoon chopped garlic

1 cup chopped onion

2 cups chopped **carrots**

2 tablespoons tomato paste

2 teaspoons kosher salt

½ tablespoon black pepper

2 teaspoons dried thyme or Herbs de Provence

6 cups chicken **stock** or low-sodium vegetable broth

Combine ingredients in a slow cooker. Cover and set on high for 8 hours. For a smoother texture, partially puree with an immersion blender before serving.

▶ **YIELD:** 8 cups

Nutrition Information per ½ Cup
Calories: 171, Total Fat: 4 grams, Saturated Fat: 1 gram, Carbohydrate: 27 grams, Sugars: 4 grams, Protein: 8 grams, Sodium: 430 milligrams, Cholesterol: 2 milligrams, Fiber: 7 grams, Vitamin D: 0 IU, Calcium: 38 milligrams, Iron: 2.5 milligrams

Grandma Lori's Baked Beans

My mom is an amazing cook, but most of her meals are created without recipes . . . just sight, smell, taste, and a lifetime of experience. This recipe was inspired by her grandmother and is now passed down to my kids. Beans are a true superfood, and yes, this recipe calls for real bacon—a little goes a long way. Forget about salty cans of baked beans; my family never has a cookout without this recipe.

2 (15-ounce) cans cannellini or pinto **beans**, rinsed and drained

2 tablespoons **maple syrup**

2 tablespoons molasses

1 teaspoon spicy yellow mustard

¼ cup ketchup

¼ teaspoon garlic salt

¼ teaspoon onion powder

2 slices bacon, cut in half

Preheat oven to 350°F. In a large bowl, combine beans, maple syrup, molasses, mustard, ketchup, garlic salt, and onion powder. Pour mixture into a baking dish and place bacon on top. Bake for 40 to 45 minutes, until beans are bubbling and bacon is crisp.

▶ **YIELD:** 3½ cups

Nutrition Information per ¼ Cup
Calories: 82, Total Fat: 1 gram, Saturated Fat: 0 grams, Carbohydrate: 15 grams, Sugars: 5 grams, Protein: 4 grams, Sodium: 100 milligrams, Cholesterol: 1 milligram, Fiber: 3 grams, Vitamin D: 1.3 IU, Calcium: 27 milligrams, Iron: 1 milligram

Slow-Cooker Pulled Pork

Pulled pork may seem like an odd suggestion for kids, but the sweet and tender pork is perfection for little eaters. This recipe makes a large batch—a must-have for Sunday football. Serve with rice, in quesadillas, or with a side of mac and cheese.

1 bulb fennel, thinly sliced

½ white onion, thinly sliced

Kosher salt and black pepper

2 tablespoons canola oil, divided

3 medium-size **pork** tenderloins (about 3 pounds), cut in half

½ cup **apple** cider or **apple** juice

½ cup barbecue sauce (Trader Joe's brand recommended)

Place fennel and onion in the bottom of a 5- to 6-quart slow cooker; season with salt and pepper. Then season pork with salt and pepper. Heat 1 tablespoon of oil in a large skillet over medium-high heat. Sear 3 pieces of the pork, cooking for about 2 minutes per side. Transfer to slow cooker on top of fennel and onion; repeat with remaining oil and pieces of pork. After removing pork, pour apple cider into hot skillet and cook for 2 minutes, using a wooden spoon to scrape any brown bits from the bottom of the pan. Pour apple cider mixture into slow cooker, followed by barbecue sauce. Cover and cook on low for 7 hours.

After 7 hours remove lid and shred pork using two forks. Add more barbecue sauce if desired. Cover and cook for 1 hour more.*

138

* If the mixture is too watery, drain some of the juices and transfer to a small saucepan; boil until it is reduced as desired and add back to slow cooker.

▶ **YIELD:** about 10 cups

Nutrition Information per 1 Cup
Calories: 130, Total Fat: 3.5 grams, Saturated Fat: 0.5 grams, Carbohydrate: 5 grams, Sugars: 3 grams, Protein: 18 grams, Sodium: 175 milligrams, Cholesterol: 55 milligrams, Fiber: 1 gram, Vitamin D: 7 IU, Calcium: 13 milligrams, Iron: 1 milligram

Grilled Turkey Cutlets

~~~~~~~~~

Chicken breast is a terrific quick and easy weeknight din-
ner, so why not do the same with turkey breast? A lean
protein and even more tender than chicken, turkey breast
can be used for fajitas, sandwiches, and stir-fries too.

   1 pound thin-sliced **turkey** breast cutlets
   ½ cup balsamic vinaigrette salad dressing

Marinate cutlets in dressing for about 30 minutes. Preheat a grill or grill pan over medium heat. Remove
meat from marinade (discard marinade) and cook for 3
to 4 minutes per side or until internal temperature
reads 160°F. Let rest for 10 minutes before slicing.

▶ **YIELD:** 5 to 6 cutlets

Nutrition Information per 2 Ounces Cooked Turkey
Calories: 81, Total Fat: 1 gram, Saturated Fat: 0 grams, Carbohydrate:
1 gram, Sugars: 1 gram, Protein: 14 grams, Sodium: 73 milligrams,
Cholesterol: 35 milligrams, Fiber: 0 grams, Vitamin D: 0 IU, Calcium:
10 milligrams, Iron: 0.7 milligrams

Homemade Peanut Butter

~~~~~~~~~~

I'm always asked what to look for in a good-quality peanut butter, and it is actually really simple—peanuts and salt! Making your own is so incredibly easy and gives you a chance to create your own signature flavors. I like to add cinnamon, honey, or unsweetened cocoa powder.

10 ounces roasted and salted **peanuts** (about 2 cups)

Place peanuts in a food processor. Pulse, then blend until peanut butter is desired consistency. Add flavorings (if using) and pulse again to combine.

▶ **YIELD:** 1 cup

Nutrition Information per 1 Tablespoon
Calories: 106, Total Fat: 9 grams, Saturated Fat: 1 gram, Carbohydrate: 3 grams, Sugars: 1 gram, Protein: 4 grams, Sodium: 72 milligrams, Cholesterol: 0 milligrams, Fiber: 1 gram, Vitamin D: 0 IU, Calcium: 0 milligrams, Iron: 0.2 milligrams

White Bean Sandwich Spread

~~~~~~~~~~

This savory spread tastes good on just about everything. Smear on a sandwich or serve with pretzels, carrots, and pita chips for dipping. This is a nice alternative to hummus and carries a lower risk of allergic reaction because it does not contain sesame seeds.

1 (15.5-ounce) can cannellini **beans**, rinsed and drained

¼ cup extra virgin olive oil

1 clove garlic

2 tablespoons whipped cream cheese

1 tablespoon fresh **lemon** juice

1½ teaspoons chopped **rosemary**

¼ teaspoon kosher salt

½ teaspoon black pepper

Add ingredients into food processor; pulse until smooth.

▶ **YIELD:** 2½ cups

Nutrition Information per ¼ Cup
Calories: 92, Total Fat: 6 grams, Saturated Fat: 1 gram, Carbohydrate: 6 grams, Sugars: 0 grams, Protein: 3 grams, Sodium: 173 milligrams, Cholesterol: 2 milligrams, Fiber: 2 grams, Vitamin D: 0 IU, Calcium: 28.33 milligrams, Iron: 0.5 milligrams

142

Panko-Breaded Fish Sticks

You'll never resort to boxed fish sticks again. Adults love them too, so make a big batch for the entire family. Greek yogurt, a little mayo, pickle relish, and fresh lemon juice make a dynamite dipping sauce.

- 1 cup all-purpose flour
- 1 **egg**, beaten with 2 tablespoons water
- 1 cup panko bread crumbs
- Kosher salt and black pepper
- 1 pound fresh **cod**, cut into 1-inch strips
- 2 tablespoons canola oil

Preheat oven to 450°F. Place a wire rack over a baking sheet and spray with nonstick spray. Set up breading station by placing flour in a resealable plastic bag, egg and water in a shallow bowl, and bread crumbs in a shallow dish; season all with salt and pepper. Dredge the pieces of fish in the flour (make sure to shake away any excess). Continue on to dip in the egg, then the bread crumb mixture. Transfer to prepared baking sheet. Drizzle with canola oil and bake for 20 to 25 minutes, until golden, turning once.

▶ **YIELD:** 10 to 12 pieces

Nutrition Information per Piece
Calories: 86, Total Fat: 3 grams, Saturated Fat: 0 grams, Carbohydrate: 6 grams, Sugars: 0 grams, Protein: 8 grams, Sodium: 79 milligrams, Cholesterol: 32 milligrams, Fiber: 0 grams, Vitamin D: 17 IU, Calcium: 8 milligrams, Iron: 0.5 milligrams

Lemon Shrimp

~~~~~~~~~

Shrimp make for a fast lean protein option when you are pressed for time to get a meal on the table. They also contain omega-3 fatty acids to help with brain development. You can serve this with green beans, pasta, or rice pilaf.

1 pound fresh **shrimp**, peeled and deveined

Juice and zest of 1 **lemon**

1 tablespoon canola oil

1 clove garlic, minced

Marinate shrimp in lemon and set aside. Heat oil in a large skillet; add garlic and sauté for 30 seconds. Add shrimp and cook for 3 to 4 minutes or until shrimp are opaque and cooked through.

▶ **YIELD:** 14 to 16 large shrimp

Nutrition Information per Shrimp
Calories: 28, Total Fat: 1 gram, Saturated Fat: 0 grams, Carbohydrate: 0 grams, Sugars: 0 grams, Protein: 4 grams, Sodium: 161 milligrams, Cholesterol: 36 milligrams, Fiber: 0 grams, Vitamin D: 1 IU, Calcium: 16 milligrams, Iron: 0 milligrams

Buzz Burgers

Sometimes all you need is a fun name to make something more appealing. Inspired by one of my kids' favorite movies, these burgers are portion-size for tiny hands but packed with muscle-building protein. Set up a burger bar at the kitchen table and let everyone pile on all their favorite fixings.

- 1 pound lean ground beef or **turkey**
- Kosher salt and black pepper
- 2 slices **American cheese**, each cut into 4 pieces
- 8 **whole wheat slider buns** or potato rolls
- Toppings: sliced tomato, lettuce, pickles, ketchup, mustard

Heat grill or grill pan to medium-high heat. Form meat into 8 burgers and season generously with salt and pepper. Cook for 4 to 5 minutes per side. Place on buns and top with cheese and desired toppings. The USDA recommendation for ground meat is 160°F to 165°F.

▶ **YIELD:** 8 burgers

Nutrition Information per Burger
Calories: 201, Total Fat: 10 grams, Saturated Fat: 4 grams, Carbohydrate: 13 grams, Sugars: 0 grams, Protein: 15 grams, Sodium: 408 milligrams, Cholesterol: 43 milligrams, Fiber: 1 gram, Vitamin D: 3 IU, Calcium: 94 milligrams, Iron: 2.3 milligrams

Crispy Chicken Fingers with Magical Honey Mustard

~~~~~~~~~

Every kid loves chicken fingers, but most frozen ones are loaded with preservatives, and the restaurant versions are drowning in grease. Using a small amount of oil and a nonstick skillet makes these fingers crispy, light, and delish. You can also bake them in a 375°F oven for 7 to 8 minutes per side. And kids love to dunk chicken in this simply magical yogurt-based sauce.

1 cup all-purpose flour

1 **egg**, beaten with a splash of water

2 cups panko bread crumbs

2 tablespoons grated **Parmesan cheese**

1¼ pounds raw **chicken** breast, cut into 14 pieces

½ cup canola oil, divided

¼ cup nonfat Greek **yogurt**

2 tablespoons yellow mustard

1 tablespoon **honey**

Set up breading station by placing flour in a resealable plastic bag, egg in a bowl, and bread crumbs mixed with Parmesan cheese in a shallow dish. Dredge the pieces of chicken in the flour (make sure to shake away any excess). Continue on to dip in the egg, then the bread crumb mixture. Heat oil in a large nonstick skillet. Cook chicken fingers in small batches for 4 minutes per side, until chicken is completely cooked. To make the dipping sauce, whisk together Greek yogurt, mustard, and honey. Serve chicken with dipping sauce on the side.

▶ **YIELD:** 14 pieces and ½ cup sauce

Nutrition Information per Serving
(2 Pieces of Chicken with 1 Tablespoon of Sauce)
Calories: 280, Total Fat: 13 grams, Saturated Fat: 2 grams, Carbohydrate: 17 grams, Sugars: 3 grams, Protein: 13 grams, Sodium: 210 milligrams, Cholesterol: 81 milligrams, Fiber: 1 gram, Vitamin D: 10 IU, Calcium: 56 milligrams, Iron: 0.9 milligrams

Roasted Salmon

~~~~~~~~~~

Seafood can be intimidating for grown-ups to cook and kids to eat. Try this recipe, and it won't be any longer. It's easy enough for a weeknight dinner but fancy enough for a holiday meal (we make it almost every Christmas Eve). Experiment with different toppings, like teriyaki, pesto, or barbecue sauce.

12 ounces wild **salmon**, skin removed, cut into 4 pieces

1 tablespoon olive oil

½ teaspoon kosher salt

2 tablespoons whole grain mustard

2 tablespoons **honey** or **maple syrup**

Lemon wedges for serving

Preheat oven to 400°F. Place salmon on a sheet pan lined with parchment paper. Drizzle with olive oil and season with salt; roast for 10 minutes. While salmon is cooking, combine mustard and honey (or maple syrup) in a small bowl. After 10 minutes of cooking, brush salmon with mustard sauce and return to the oven for an additional 5 to 7 minutes or until salmon is cooked through. Serve with a squeeze of fresh lemon juice.

▶ **YIELD:** 4 pieces

Nutrition Information per Piece (About 2½ Ounces)
Calories: 168, Total Fat: 8 grams, Saturated Fat: 1 gram, Carbohydrate: 5 grams, Sugars: 4 grams, Protein: 19 grams, Sodium: 250 milligrams, Cholesterol: 49 milligrams, Fiber: 0 grams, Vitamin D: 0 IU, Calcium: 5 milligrams, Iron: 0.5 milligrams

6

Dairy and Egg Recipes

· 6 TO 12 MONTHS ·

Peach-Swirl Yogurt

Many popular brands of yogurt marketed to kids are loaded with processed sweeteners and artificial colors. To avoid all the junk, consider using plain yogurt and adding your own flavors whenever you can. Greek yogurt is higher in protein and lower in lactose for sensitive tummies, and all yogurts contain probiotics for a healthy digestive system. Stock up on homemade peach preserves on your next trip to the local farmers' market.

1 cup plain nonfat Greek **yogurt**

1 teaspoon **peach** preserves or fruit spread

2 tablespoons freshly squeezed **orange** juice

Combine ingredients in a medium bowl and whisk to combine.

▶ **YIELD:** about 1¼ cups

Nutrition Information per ¼ Cup
Calories: 38, Total Fat: 0 grams, Saturated Fat: 0 grams, Carbohydrate: 4 grams, Sugars: 4 grams, Protein: 5 grams, Sodium: 22 milligrams, Cholesterol: 0 milligrams, Fiber: 0 grams, Vitamin D: 0 IU, Calcium: 64 milligrams, Iron: 0 milligrams

Spoonable Smoothie

~~~~~~

Infants can't really handle using a straw, but this thick and creamy smoothie can be enjoyed by the tiny spoon-ful. Make this with any type of fruit; infants love mango, banana, and peaches.

1 cup frozen fruit (**bananas**, **berries**, **peaches**, **pineapple**)

1 cup boxed **coconut** milk

Combine ingredients in a blender and blend until smooth.

▶ **YIELD:** 1½ cups

Nutrition Information per ¼ Cup
Calories: 30, Total Fat: 1 gram, Saturated Fat: 1 gram, Carbohydrate: 6 grams, Sugars: 5 grams, Protein: 0 grams, Sodium: 3 milligrams, Cholesterol: 0 milligrams, Fiber: 1 gram, Vitamin D: 20 IU, Calcium: 5 milligrams, Iron: 0.2 milligrams

Veggie Scramble

~~~~~~~~

Chop veggies extra small and add a sprinkle of cheese for a rainbow-colored breakfast in minutes. Eggs are one of the best protein options you can find, plus yolks are filled with antioxidants like lutein for eyesight and omega-3 fats for a healthy brain.

2 large **eggs**

Kosher salt and black pepper

½ cup chopped vegetables (**bell pepper**, **broccoli**, **spinach**, mushrooms)

2 tablespoons shredded **cheese**

Heat a small nonstick skillet over medium heat and spray with nonstick cooking spray. In a small bowl, whisk eggs and season with salt and pepper. Add eggs and vegetables to pan and scramble for about 1 minute. Add cheese and continue to gently scramble until eggs are fluffy and cheese is melted.

▶ **YIELD:** 2 servings

Nutrition Information per Serving
Calories: 96, Total Fat: 6 grams, Saturated Fat: 2 grams, Carbohydrate: 1 gram, Sugars: 1 gram, Protein: 9 grams, Sodium: 130 milligrams, Cholesterol: 190 milligrams, Fiber: 0.5 grams, Vitamin D: 41 IU, Calcium: 84 milligrams, Iron: 1 milligram

Nonni's Chocolate Pudding

~~~~~~~~~~

I was raised on my grandmother's chocolate pudding, and it is an honor to make it for my girls. Make this pudding for a calcium-filled dessert all by itself or make trifle, icebox cake, pudding pops, and other goodies.

2 cups whole **milk**

1 tablespoon unsalted butter

5 tablespoons sugar

2 tablespoons unsweetened **cocoa** powder

2 tablespoons cornstarch

2 tablespoons water

1 teaspoon pure vanilla or almond extract

In a medium saucepan, combine milk and butter. Heat over medium-low heat, stirring gently to melt butter. In a small bowl, combine sugar, cocoa, and cornstarch—add water and mix to create a paste. Add paste into milk mixture and whisk well to combine. Raise heat to medium and cook, stirring with a wooden spoon until thick and bubbly (about 5 minutes). Remove from heat and stir in extract. Transfer to a bowl or 4 ramekins, cover with plastic wrap (make sure plastic is touching pudding to prevent a skin from forming), and refrigerate for at least 4 hours.

▶ **YIELD:** 2½ cups

153

Nutrition Information per ½ Cup
Calories: 148, Total Fat: 6 grams, Saturated Fat: 3 grams, Carbohydrate: 21 grams, Sugars: 18 grams, Protein: 3 grams, Sodium: 43 milligrams, Cholesterol: 16 milligrams, Fiber: 1 gram, Vitamin D: 3.65 IU, Calcium: 114 milligrams, Iron: 0.33 milligrams

Lemon-Ricotta Cookies

~~~~~~

A holiday favorite, these cookies are a twist on a traditional Italian cookie. These lemony delights are light as air but super flavorful and not overpowering in any way. You can also make the dough ahead and freeze— scoop a ball of dough (using a mini ice-cream scoop) onto a sheet pan and place in the freezer until hardened, then place in a freezer-safe bag. When ready to bake, do not thaw. Place directly in a preheated oven and increase the cooking time by 1 to 2 minutes.

½ cup all-purpose flour

½ cup **whole wheat pastry flour**

½ teaspoon baking powder

¾ teaspoon kosher salt

½ cup unsalted butter

1 cup granulated sugar

1 large **egg**

1 teaspoon vanilla extract

1 cup whole milk **ricotta cheese**

2 teaspoons grated **lemon** zest

FOR THE GLAZE

1 cup confectioners' sugar

2 teaspoons freshly squeezed **lemon** juice

1 tablespoon whole **milk**

Sprinkles or other cookie decorations (optional)

Line a baking sheet with parchment paper or Silpat and set aside. Preheat oven to 350°F.

In a large bowl, sift together flours, baking powder, and salt; set aside. In a stand mixer fitted with a paddle attachment cream together the butter and sugar. With the mixer on low, add the egg, followed by vanilla extract, ricotta, and lemon zest. Slowly add the flour mixture to the mixer and mix on low until all the flour is incorporated. Spoon tablespoons of dough onto prepared baking sheet (leave at least 2 inches between cookies, they spread a lot!). Bake 1 dozen cookies at a time for 10 to 12 minutes, until the bottoms are golden brown (the tops will remain pale yellow). Cool for 10 minutes, then transfer to a wire rack to cool completely. While remaining batches are baking and cooling, prepare the glaze.

In a small bowl, whisk together confectioners' sugar, lemon juice, and milk. Glaze should have a loose consistency but should still coat the back of a spoon. Spoon about ½ teaspoon of glaze onto each cookie and allow to drip off the sides. Sprinkle with desired decorations and allow to set for at least 20 minutes (you can speed this up by placing in the refrigerator).

▶ **YIELD:** 36 cookies

Nutrition Information per Cookie
Calories: 84, Total Fat: 4 grams, Saturated Fat: 2 grams, Carbohydrate: 12 grams, Sugars: 9 grams, Protein: 1 gram, Sodium: 38 milligrams, Cholesterol: 15 milligrams, Fiber: 0 grams, Vitamin D: 4 IU, Calcium: 18 milligrams, Iron: 0.2 milligrams

Vanilla Bean Frozen Yogurt

~~~~~~~

There's nothing better on a summer day than a home-made frozen treat. Instead of dealing with complicated ice-cream recipes, I like to toss some yogurt in the machine—it's higher in protein and an excellent source of tummy-pleasing probiotics.

⅓ cup superfine sugar

Seeds of 1 vanilla bean

1½ cups reduced-fat (2 percent) Greek **yogurt**

½ cup low-fat vanilla **yogurt**

In a large bowl, whisk sugar, vanilla, and yogurts and transfer to an ice-cream maker. Mix according to the manufacturer's suggestions, until thick and frosty (10–15 minutes). Enjoy immediately, or transfer to a freezer-safe container and allow to harden in the freezer for 1 hour. Store in the freezer for up to 1 week.

Variation

For a fruit-flavored yogurt: In a small saucepan, combine 2 cups of fresh fruit and ½ cup sugar over medium heat. Bring to a simmer and cook for 15 minutes until thickened—set aside to cool completely. In a large bowl, whisk yogurts together with cooled fruit mixture, then transfer to an ice-cream maker.

156

▶ **YIELD:** about 2½ cups

Nutrition Information per ½ Cup
Calories: 109, Total Fat: 0 grams, Saturated Fat: 0 grams, Carbohydrate: 19 grams, Sugars: 19 grams, Protein: 8 grams, Sodium: 43 milligrams, Cholesterol: 1 milligram, Fiber: 0 grams, Vitamin D: 0.25 IU, Calcium: 132.59 milligrams, Iron: 0.2 milligrams

Hot Chocolate

~~~~~~~~

A cozy cup of hot cocoa is perfect for a winter night, plus the extra dose of calcium and vitamin D is just what the doctor ordered for growing bones. Agave dissolves nicely and is sweeter than sugar, so you can use less. Since a big mug of warm liquid may not be the best idea for younger kids, serve gently warmed with a straw or a spoon—it also works in a sippy cup.

2 cups whole **milk**

2 tablespoons agave nectar

2 tablespoons unsweetened **cocoa** powder

Place ingredients in a small saucepan; whisk well. Heat over medium-high heat, whisking occasionally until hot and frothy.

▶ **YIELD:** 2 cups

Nutrition Information per ½ Cup
Calories: 113, Total Fat: 5 grams, Saturated Fat: 3 grams, Carbohydrate: 16 grams, Sugars: 14 grams, Protein: 5 grams, Sodium: 63 milligrams, Cholesterol: 18 milligrams, Fiber: 1 gram, Vitamin D: 50 IU, Calcium: 150 milligrams, Iron: 0.72 milligrams

Turkey and Cheese Panini

~~~~~~~~~~

Take a break from boring grilled cheese. This pressed sandwich has a boost of flavor and protein from turkey breast. To make this sandwich even more special, pick up some bakery-fresh whole grain bread. Cut into triangles for older kids and into small bite-size pieces for little ones.

2 slices **whole grain bread**

Buttery spread such as Smart Balance

2 slices **cheddar** or **American cheese**

2 ounces sliced **turkey** breast (such as Applegate)

Preheat panini press or nonstick skillet. Arrange one slice of bread on a flat surface; cover evenly with spread and turn over. Top nonbuttered side of bread with a piece of cheese followed by turkey. Top with additional slice of cheese and bread, then coat that piece with buttery spread. Transfer to pan and cook for about 3 minutes per side or until bread is golden and cheese is melted.

▶ **YIELD:** 1 sandwich

Nutrition Information per ¼ Sandwich
Calories: 113, Total Fat: 6 grams, Saturated Fat: 3 grams, Carbohydrate: 11 grams, Sugars: 2 grams, Protein: 5 grams, Sodium: 316 milligrams, Cholesterol: 12 milligrams, Fiber: 2 grams, Vitamin D: 10 IU, Calcium: 67 milligrams, Iron: 0.6 milligrams

Paris-Inspired Omelet

~~~~~~~~~~

This omelet's name is derived from one of our favorite movies, Disney's Ratatouille. *Once I suggested "Let's make an omelet like Remy does," the kids were sold. We make it with basil (just like in the movie), but anything goes!*

2 large **eggs**

1 tablespoon water

Kosher salt and black pepper

1 tablespoon chopped fresh **basil**

1 ounce shredded **cheese**

Heat a nonstick skillet over medium heat. Combine eggs and water in a bowl, season with salt and pepper to taste, and whisk well. Add basil to egg mixture. Spray a nonstick skillet with nonstick cooking spray. Add eggs and cook for 2 to 3 minutes, until eggs begin to set. Using a spatula, gently pull in the sides of the omelet to let the uncooked egg run to the edges of the pan. Sprinkle cheese evenly on top and gently fold in half. Allow to cook for 2 to 3 more minutes, until eggs are completely set and cheese is melted.

▶ **YIELD:** 2 servings

Nutrition Information per Serving
Calories: 73, Total Fat: 5 grams, Saturated Fat: 3 grams, Carbohydrate: 1 gram, Sugars: 0 grams, Protein: 7 grams, Sodium: 226 milligrams, Cholesterol: 13 milligrams, Fiber: 0 grams, Vitamin D: 0 IU, Calcium: 106 milligrams, Iron: 0.2 milligrams

Egg Salad Sliders

Packed with antioxidants like lutein plus additional nutrients like protein and healthy fats, these tasty sliders are a healthy twist on tea sandwiches. An added bonus, the soft texture makes them easy to chew. For perfect hard-boiled eggs, place eggs in a saucepan and cover with cool water. Heat on high until water boils. Once boiling, turn off heat, cover, and allow to sit for 15 minutes; drain and cool. Try this recipe with canned tuna instead of eggs for a killer tuna salad.

- 2 hard-boiled **eggs**, finely chopped
- 1 tablespoon mayonnaise
- 1 tablespoon nonfat Greek **yogurt**
- 2 tablespoons shredded **carrots**
- 2 tablespoons finely chopped celery
- 1 tablespoon chopped **chives**
- ¼ teaspoon kosher salt
- ¼ teaspoon paprika (optional)
- 4 mini potato or **whole wheat dinner rolls**

In a bowl, combine eggs, mayo, and yogurt; mash with a fork until combined. Fold in carrots, celery, chives, and spices. Serve on rolls.

▶ **YIELD:** 4 sandwiches

Nutrition Information per 1 Sandwich
Calories: 138, Total Fat: 7 grams, Saturated Fat: 2 grams, Carbohydrate: 14 grams, Sugars: 1 gram, Protein: 6 grams, Sodium: 265 milligrams, Cholesterol: 94 milligrams, Fiber: 1 gram, Vitamin D: 21 IU, Calcium: 71 milligrams, Iron: 1.5 milligrams

Maddy's Special Egg Sandwich

My oldest went through a "no yellow" phase, and instead of giving up on eggs altogether, we temporarily skipped the yolks for this breakfast sandwich. Occasionally we would add some turkey bacon too. I hate wasting anything, so I save the yolks to make hollandaise sauce.

1 large **egg** white

Pinch of kosher salt

Black pepper

1 slice **white cheddar** or **American cheese**

1 **whole grain English muffin**, split and toasted

Heat a small nonstick skillet over medium heat and spray with nonstick spray. Place egg white in a bowl; scramble with a fork and season with salt and pepper to taste. Pour egg white into skillet and gently scramble. Once cooked through, turn off heat and top egg with cheese until slightly melted. Assemble sandwich on muffin and serve.

▶ **YIELD:** 1 sandwich

Nutrition Information per Sandwich
Calories: 212, Total Fat: 8 grams, Saturated Fat: 5 grams, Carbohydrate: 19 grams, Sugars: 2 grams, Protein: 14 grams, Sodium: 530 milligrams, Cholesterol: 19 milligrams, Fiber: 3 grams, Vitamin D: 0 IU, Calcium: 195 milligrams, Iron: 0.2 milligrams

Ham, Cheddar, and Basil Quiche Cups

~~~~~~~~~

Motherhood has taught me that everything tastes better when made in a cupcake tin. This recipe is even more of a winner when we frame it as my take on "green eggs and ham." These delectable high-protein finger foods are also a wonderful addition to a brunch menu for grown-ups.

7 large **eggs**

½ cup half-and-half

¼ cup fresh **basil** leaves

½ teaspoon kosher salt

Black pepper

1 refrigerated pie crust

2 ounces deli **ham**, finely chopped

3 ounces shredded **cheddar cheese**

Preheat oven to 350°F. Add eggs, half-and-half, and basil to blender; season with salt and pepper to taste and blend to combine. Roll out pie dough and, using a paring knife or ring mold, cut out 12 circles (you will have some dough left over). Place 1 circle of dough at the bottom of each cup in a cupcake tin. Pour egg mixture on top, filling each muffin cup about two-thirds of the way full. Add some ham and cheese to each and bake for 15 minutes or until eggs are set. Remove from the oven and allow to cool for at least 15 minutes before serving.

162

▶ **YIELD:** 12 pieces

Nutrition Information per Piece
Calories: 129, Total Fat: 9 grams, Saturated Fat: 4 grams, Carbohydrate: 6 grams, Sugars: 0 grams, Protein: 7 grams, Sodium: 220 milligrams, Cholesterol: 124 milligrams, Fiber: 0 grams, Vitamin D: 26 IU, Calcium: 79 milligrams, Iron: 0.6 milligrams

Yogurt Sundaes

~~~~~~~~~~

The yogurt section of the grocery store can be incredibly overwhelming! So much to choose from and so much of it is high-sugar junk. It's fine to resort to a good-quality presweetened yogurt for lunch boxes and meals on the go, but when I have the time I love to set up a yogurt bar. I start with plain yogurt, and the kids get to choose from all kinds of healthy toppings.

1½ cups plain nonfat Greek **yogurt**

2 teaspoons ground flaxseed

½ cup granola or **whole grain cereal**

1 cup chopped fresh fruit (**berries, pears, bananas, melon**)

Honey or **maple syrup**

Layer ingredients in a serving glass, alternating yogurt, flaxseed, granola, and berries. Drizzle with honey (or maple syrup) and serve.

▶ **YIELD:** 3 cups

Nutrition Information per ½ Cup
Calories: 84, Total Fat: 1 gram, Saturated Fat: 0 grams, Carbohydrate: 13 grams, Sugars: 6 grams, Protein: 6 grams, Sodium: 22 milligrams, Cholesterol: 0 milligrams, Fiber: 2 grams, Vitamin D: 20 IU, Calcium: 68 milligrams, Iron: 0.4 milligrams

Tropical Milk Shake

~~~~~~~~

This shake is loaded with extra calcium and vitamin D from yogurt plus fortified OJ. Make extra and freeze leftovers in ice pop molds.

1 cup frozen mango chunks

1 small container (5–6 ounces) coconut-flavored Greek **yogurt** (Chobani brand recommended)

1 cup calcium-fortified **orange** juice

Combine ingredients in a blender and blend until smooth.

▶ **YIELD:** about 3 cups

Nutrition Information per 1 Cup
Calories: 120, Total Fat: 2 grams, Saturated Fat: 1 gram, Carbohydrate: 22 grams, Sugars: 19 grams, Protein: 5 grams, Sodium: 21 milligrams, Cholesterol: 5 milligrams, Fiber: 1 gram, Vitamin D: 33 IU, Calcium: 173 milligrams, Iron: 0.1 milligrams

7

Ten Healthy Kid-Friendly Menus

I n an effort to help parents answer the age-old question "What should I make?" here are ten easy ideas for various occasions. Most are best for children ages eighteen months and up but can be modified as needed. Recipes that appear in this book include page numbers.

WEEKDAY BREAKFAST
- Cinnamon Roll Oatmeal (page 122)
- Fresh fruit

WEEKEND BREAKFAST
- Whole Grain Pancakes (page 100)
- Peach-Swirl Yogurt (page 149)

LUNCH FOR A BUNCH
- Guac for All Ages (page 61)
- Vegetable and Black Bean Quesadillas (page 77)
- Clementine Dippers (page 96)

FAMILY MOVIE NIGHT

- *Real* Microwave Popcorn (page 123)
- Crispy Chicken Fingers with Magical Honey Mustard (page 146)
- Cucumbers with Homemade Ranch Dressing (page 90)
- Vanilla Bean Frozen Yogurt (page 156)

MOTHER'S DAY BRUNCH

- Ham, Cheddar, and Basil Quiche Cups (page 162)
- Blueberry–Greek Yogurt Mini Muffins (page 104)
- Freshly squeezed OJ

FATHER'S DAY COOKOUT

- Buzz Burgers (page 145)
- Veggie Kebabs (page 94)
- Grandma Lori's Baked Beans (page 137)
- Sliced watermelon

BEACH PICNIC

- Watermelon-Pineapple-Carrot Juice (page 75)
- Homemade Peanut Butter (page 141) and jelly sandwiches
- Whole wheat pretzels

DINNER PLAYDATE

- Grilled Turkey Cutlets (page 140)
- Green Beans with Homemade French Dressing (page 76)
- Whole grain bread
- Fruit-Burst Ice Pops (page 87)

HOLIDAY DINNER

- Roasted Salmon (page 148)
- Roasted Root Vegetables (page 92)
- Lemon-Ricotta Cookies (page 154)

BIRTHDAY CELEBRATION

- Three-Cheese Pizza (page 106)
- Veggie platter
- Whole Grain Chocolate Cupcakes with Cream Cheese and Mascarpone Frosting (page 109)

Acknowledgments

I am so incredibly fortunate for all the enthusiasm, guidance, and support I have received as I worked tirelessly to make this book happen.

First and foremost, my family. Special thanks to my brother Chris for learning to cook alongside me and for still challenging me to cook-offs. To my mother and father, Lori and Bobby, for raising us kids to love real food, and to my "Nonni" Lillian for teaching all of us to appreciate the beauty of a family recipe. To my husband, Zack, for tolerating my work ethic, growing with me, and inspiring me to create (no matter how badly I trash the kitchen). To my spectacular daughters, Madeline and Charlotte, for making me smile every day and for (almost) always being willing to try new things.

A special thank-you to Dalyn Miller and Holly Schmidt from Holland Publishing for sparking the fire for *First Bites*, and to the amazing editorial team at Perigee and the Penguin Group, particularly Jeanette Shaw, who provided much-needed guidance for a newbie cookbook author.

I would not be where I am today if it wasn't for my graduate school education, the faculty at Teachers College, Columbia University, including Joan Gussow, who taught me to value where food comes from, and Lora Sporny, who introduced me to the important facets of feeding children, and the brilliant work of Ellyn Satter.

There are also countless colleagues and friends that helped make this book possible.

Amazing fellow RDs Toby Amidor, Jenna Bell, and Kyle Shadix, who fostered my love of culinary nutrition from the very beginning. To Devan Alusik for always being up to a recipe challenge, and to my local farmer Lexi Gazy for providing the freshest ingredients. To Andie and Ilisa for being the outlets for my overtired and stressed-out rants. To a team of amazing neighborhood moms for their encouragement and conversation, and to Jess and Jenny for their willingness to get their hands dirty testing recipes. I am forever grateful and look forward to watching our children grow together.

Index

~~~~~~~~

Page numbers in **bold** indicate tables; those in *italics* indicate recipes.

175

176

177

About the Author

Dana Angelo White, MS, RD, ATC, is a registered dietitian, certified athletic trainer, nutrition and fitness consultant, and mother to a three-year-old and a five-year-old. She specializes in culinary nutrition for children and adults, recipe development, and sports nutrition.

Dana works closely with chefs and authors to develop creative and healthy recipes for cookbooks, magazines, and menus. She is the nutrition expert for FoodNetwork.com and founding contributor for Food Network's *Healthy Eats* blog. She has worked as the nutrition consultant for Follow Productions on seasons 2 and 3 of Bobby Deen's show *Not My Mama's Meals*. She has worked as a media spokesperson for *Cooking Light* and has made appearances on *Good Day Street Talk*, FoodNetwork.com, *Access Hollywood*, and *Good Morning America Health*. In October 2013, Dana was named to Sharecare's list of Top 10 Social Health-Makers on Nutrition.

Dana is an assistant clinical faculty member and sports dietitian at Quinnipiac University in Hamden, Connecticut. She also conducts workshops and cooking demonstrations for fitness organizations and schools from preschool to college.

179

Dana's recipes and articles have been featured on FoodNetwork.com, CookingLight.com, DietTV.com, *Today's Dietitian, Shape, Seventeen, Maxim,* and *Prevention.* She has created meal plans and recipes for books including *Energy to Burn: The Ultimate Food and Nutrition Guide to Fuel Your Active Life* (2009), *Tell Me What to Eat If I Am Trying to Conceive: Nutrition You Can Live With* (2011), *Extra Lean: The Fat-Burning Plan That Changes the Way You Eat for Life* (2011), *Extra Lean Family: Get Lean and Achieve Your Family's Best Health Ever* (2012) by Mario Lopez, and *The PrayFit Diet* (2014) by Jimmy Peña and Eric Velazquez.

A farmers' market junkie and local food aficionado, Dana worked with Harvard Medical School's Center for Health and the Global Environment to create the Healthy Harvest regional food guides to educate consumers on purchasing and preparing seasonal foods.

Dana has spent the last several years raising her two daughters. She has immersed herself in cooking and creating recipes for them to devour while finding inspiration from fellow parents and her backyard garden.

Dana earned her master's degree in nutrition education from Teachers College, Columbia University, and her bachelor's degree in sports medicine from Quinnipiac University. She lives in Fairfield, Connecticut, with her husband, children, and terrier, Violet Pickles.